YOUR BIRTH PLAN

Creating *your* path
for a fulfilling pregnancy, birth
and postpartum journey

Kathy M. Stewart, RN, CPNP, IBCLC,
LCCE, CD Trainer (DONA)

Your Birth Plan

Kathy M. Stewart

ISBN: 978-1-936553-06-8

PLEASE NOTE:
This book is meant to be a guide for writing your birth plan and not a substitute for asking and receiving medical advice and prenatal care from a healthcare provider.
Your pregnancy is unique and you may experience obstetrical needs beyond the scope of this book.
Going to regularly scheduled prenatal and postpartum visits are vital for the health and safety of you and your baby.

Cover by Designer Rob Sheley, Richmond, VA
CD Music by Joshua Seolaro
Recorded at The Basement, Richmond, VA

Warwick House Publishers
720 Court Street
Lynchburg, Virginia 24504

This book is dedicated to:

My two sons, Bradford and Adam—
you give me more love, joy and laughter in life
than you will ever know.
My life is blessed every day by having
you two as my sons.

My parents, Russell and Rachel Malone,
for providing a Christian home filled with love and laughter
while teaching my sister, brother and me many life lessons.
Mom, a special thank you for teaching me that birth was
a positive experience, always saying birth was short and easy.
You are one strong woman. Love you.

Contents

Acknowledgments ix

Introduction 1

Chapter One: Journey of Discovery 3
- Your Mindset for Pregnancy 5
- So, What's Next? 7
- Developing the "I can handle it" Attitude 8
- Getting Yourself to the Next Level of Belief 8
- Positive Thinking 8
- Heighten Your Awareness 11
- Relaxation Techniques 13

Chapter Two: Your Birth Plan 21
- Your Mindset for Birth 22
- How Do You Change Your Subconscious Mind? 25
- Writing Your Birth Plan 27
- Stress, Pain, and Catecholamines 32
- Doula Support 34

Chapter Three: Labor and Birth 37
- Anatomy and Physiology 37
- Warning Signs During Late Pregnancy 40
- The Four Stages of Labor 41
  - Phase One—Latent or Early Labor 42
    - How to Time and Evaluate a Contraction 43
    - When to Call Your Doctor or Midwife 45
    - What to Bring to the Hospital 45
    - Hospital Bag 47
    - During Early Labor 51
  - Phase Two—Active Labor 53
    - During Active Labor 54

Phase Three—Transitional Labor 56
During Transitional Labor 57
The Second Stage of Labor 58
Let the Pushing Begin! 58
During the Second Stage of Labor 59
The Third Stage of Labor 63
During the Third Stage of Labor 63
The Fourth Stage of Labor 64
During the Fourth Stage of Labor 64
Interventions 65
Electronic Fetal Monitoring 65
Intravenous Fluids 65
Pitocin 66
Amniotomy 66
Medically Assisted Births 67
Use of Forceps 67
Vacuum Extractor 67
Episiotomy 67
Medications During Labor 68
Analgesics 68
Epidural Anesthesia 68
Local Anesthesia 70
When a Caesarean Birth Becomes Necessary 70

Chapter Four: Postpartum 75
Your Mindset for Postpartum 76
Your Hospital Stay 80
The Newborn 80
Bonding 81
Characteristics of Your Newborn 82
The Measurements and What They Mean 87
Postpartum for Mom 90
Postpartum Depression 92

Chapter Five: Parenthood 95
Your Mindset on Becoming a Parent 96
Birth Stories 98
Austin's Birth Story 98
Baby Ellie's Birth Story 102
Wyatt's Birth Story 105
Carson's Birth Story 112
Maeve's Birth Story—Labor of Love 114
Kaysen, Henley and Louisa's Birth Stories 116
Lula's Birth Story 121
Asher's Birth Story 127
Evan's Birth Story 129
James' Birth Story 132
Reagan's Birth Story 134
Liberty "Libby" Grace's Birth Story 136
Owen's Birth Story 138
Jasper's Birth Story 140
Sabine and Simone's Birth Stories 143
Elena Ivy's Birth Story 147
Lucian's Birth Story 151
20 Things That Matter in Life 155

In Summary 157

References 159

Journal Pages 160

Sample Birth Plan Card 164

Glossary 167

Recommended Reading 173

About the Author 175

Acknowledgments

For anyone that I ever had a conversation with concerning birth, postpartum, breastfeeding or parenthood, you have influenced my decision for writing this book. It was your continuous encouragement that motivated me to get started. From the first to the final chapter, your experiences gave me important lessons that needed to be written and shared. I may not remember all of your names but if we have met and shared a story, thank you.

I must start with a huge thank you to my editor and friend, Jamie Fueglein and his wife, Karla Helbert. Our first meeting was when their son, Theo, was born and was brought to my office for his weight check. We immediately connected and enjoyed talking at each monthly office visit. Sadly, Theo was diagnosed with a rare brain tumor and died at nine months of age. Several years later, I had the privilege of being the doula at their daughter, Lula's, birth. Again, at one of the frequent and fun monthly well checkup visits, I mentioned my book writing adventure. Jamie is a professor in the English Department at Virginia Commonwealth University. I asked him about editing. I was thrilled when he agreed to help me. So, here I am, book completed, edited and ready for the publisher. I couldn't have done it without Jamie's help and his patience. Karla's input was invaluable. Thank you.

My dear friend, Jim Adair, I want to thank you for all the encouragement you gave me in writing this book, for the quiet, relaxing retreat at Lake Gaston, Virginia, and for the joy you have brought back into my life. During those days when life got busy, you kept me focused on my goal of finishing my first book. I will always be grateful.

From the book publishing to the recording of the CD, I wish to thank the individuals involved in this process. I couldn't have done it without everyone's expertise and guidance. My working relationship with all of you will always be appreciated and remembered.

Joyce Maddox and Amy Moore of Warwick House Publishers, your hours of hard work with editing, formatting and proofing were so valuable, along your patience with my many questions. The quality of the finished book shows your eye for detail.

Rob Sheley, working with you in designing the cover has been my pleasure. I had a vision, and your suggestions and creative talent moved me to love the finished look.

Joshua Seolaro, you made the most stressful part for me, recording the CD, into an enjoyable and positive experience with your easygoing manner and encouraging words. I can't thank you enough.

Molly Harrison, it has been exciting watching you and your sister grow up to become beautiful young ladies. Even though your anatomy sketches are a small view of your work, you are an excellent artist. I wish you the best in the future.

I would like to acknowledge photographers Meghan McSweeney and Jody Gillis of Photography by Jody for their contributions of several professional photographs.

I wish to thank all the couples that have attended my Lamaze classes over the past twenty-five years and who have enjoyed all my humor while learning comfort measures and skills for birthing. I have loved every moment.

I have been touched and blessed by the couples that have given me the honor of being present at the births of your children. Thank you for giving me the privilege of witnessing some of life's simple joys and blessings as I watched you become a family. Each birth holds a special place in my heart and adds inspiration in writing this book.

I need to praise and support my doula friends who understand the importance of physical and emotional support to couples during the labor, birth and postpartum periods as you help them begin their transition into parenthood. If our devoted continuous support allows a woman to feel empowered, exhilarated and self-confident after tackling the challenges of labor, we have done our job. Keep up the dedicated work.

A very special thank you to Penny Simkin for being a friend and mentor. You changed my life in 1996 after attending my first birth doula workshop. Your work has touched more women than you will ever know. Thanks from the bottom of my heart.

YOUR BIRTH PLAN

Creating *your* path
for a fulfilling pregnancy, birth
and postpartum journey

Introduction

Your birth journey is about to begin and I want you to start it with an open mind, an open heart and open arms in order to embrace all that is happening to you. Birth is overwhelming, but in a positive way, just by the sheer amazement of your body's ability to conceive, grow and birth your baby. You will always remember, especially during quiet moments, the enchantment and awe of feeling your baby's movements and kicks. This also holds true for your partner as he/she sees or feels the baby move when their hands are on your belly.

The first goal of this book is to help you examine the many physical and emotional changes and to help you enhance your birth experience as you travel this journey. This book is written in a format that will discuss a topic and encourage you to think about your mindset as it presently is. Hopefully, you will broaden your thinking and set new goals, wishes and desires. This is fun for both partners. I like for couples to keep a journal of thoughts and feelings of the pregnancy, information from each doctor's visit, and plans for the birth. For this reason, you'll find a section in the back of this book with blank journal pages on which you may write. Writing down feelings and ideas can help sort any fears that may be present due to misinformation, as well as helping you organize your desires in order to plan for a positive birth experience. Your feelings and ideas may change after you attend childbirth classes or read materials on pregnancy and birth. This growth through knowledge will move you to the next level of confidence. This confidence will empower you and your partner to embrace the magnitude of the miracle of your growing baby, birthing your baby, and then parenting this little one.

A second goal of this book is to teach you ways to use many of these techniques in your everyday life. You will learn how to visualize what it is you want, and perhaps develop some helpful habits for successful living. You will learn that attitude is a choice, how gratitude puts meaning into life, and how appreciation for our loved ones makes us kind, thankful, and loving people. This birth is just one of life's transitions that brings along with it challenges, successes, love, and much laughter.

While reading this book, if you find yourself staring out of the window, remembering your childhood, daydreaming of the future with your baby and visualizing ways of becoming a good parent, I feel I have accomplished another one of my goals for you. This book is about expanding your thinking and encouraging you to visualize goals, remembering always to live life every day to the fullest.

CHAPTER ONE
Journey of Discovery

So, you are pregnant or are planning to become pregnant. Congratulations! Becoming a parent is a wonderful part of life. Your days will be filled with unconditional love and joy beyond your imagination. Your world will expand with laughter, smiles, memories, picture taking, play groups, music lessons, sporting events, holiday traditions and family bonding times. Now, I don't wish to sugarcoat it. Yes, you may experience some nights (weeks, years) of sleep deprivation, hours of worrying about your parenting skills and receive unsolicited advice from well-meaning family members, friends and even strangers. You may think only the early months of parenthood will be hectic, but it's not until your child drives your car by herself for the first time that you realize nighttime feedings and sleep deprivation don't seem all that bad.

Giving birth is a journey of discovery—a discovery of one's abilities, of building confidence, of embracing fears, of experiencing nature at the basic level, of sharing emotional and spiritual bonding with your partner and of understanding the magnitude and privilege of being a parent to this new precious baby. Pregnancy and birth is a period in a woman's life when she may become acutely aware of the emotional and physical changes of her body and of relationship changes with her partner, family and friends. She is about to learn the strong, intuitive protective mechanism that she will display if anyone even thinks of harming her baby.

You will start discovering your abilities by keeping your body strong and healthy for your growing baby. Think about this: you have new life growing inside you. Your baby's organs develop during those first few weeks after conception. Seek medical care. Take prenatal vitamins. Eat fruits, vegetables and proteins, and go easy on processed foods, sweets, sodas, candies, empty calories food or any type of "diet" foods. Exercise can be fun. Just walk twenty to thirty minutes a day. If you like to go to the gym, check with your healthcare provider, whether she is a doctor, midwife or nurse practitioner. She will usually encourage you to keep up your exercise routine. Besides walking, another excellent form of exercise is prenatal yoga. This conditions and strengthens your body, and will teach you different poses as well as breathing and relaxation techniques to enhance your labor. It's also a great way to meet other pregnant women who share a common bond. This weekly meeting feeds your emotional side. Your physical and emotional wellness is crucial for your growing baby's health. As shown in a recent study headed by Dr. Miguel Diego and published in *Psychosomatic Medicine*, "the fetuses of mothers with higher rates of depression, anxiety and stress weighed less and were smaller than average."

Now it's time to begin to examine your mindset—your thoughts and feelings—about pregnancy and birth. Your beliefs will affect the choices you make about your upcoming birth. Let's start with pregnancy. What is your mindset about pregnancy? What is your present thinking? Is it positive or negative? What are your feelings about body changes, frequent doctor visits, watching your diet? What is your attitude about the role changes that will take place as you become a mother?

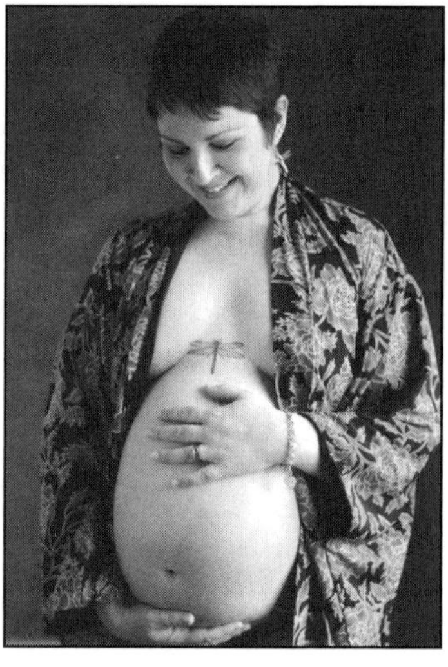

Love your body as your baby grows. Photo owned by Meghan McSweeney

Feel free to flip to the blank journal pages in the back of this book to use for this exercise. This "Your Mindset for Pregnancy" exercise can be done by you and your partner together or separately. It can help reveal the attitudes you and your partner hold, as well as to help you recognize where you each stand on pregnancy issues. Use it as a tool for communication and sharing. Doing this exercise early in the pregnancy gives each of you time to read, learn, understand and grow together.

Once you realize your body's amazing ability to grow and birth your baby, and your partner realizes his important role to love, protect and support you during this time, you both will always appreciate the closeness and bond that develops between you.

Your Mindset for Pregnancy

1. List three feelings you had when you first discovered you were pregnant.
   a. ______________________________
   b. ______________________________
   c. ______________________________

2. List three goals you set for yourself regarding this pregnancy.
   a. ______________________________
   b. ______________________________
   c. ______________________________

3. What was your partner's reaction to this pregnancy?

   ____

   ____

4. Who was the second person you called about the exciting news and why?

   ____

   ____

5. Who will you choose for your healthcare provider? (midwife or doctor)

   ____

6. Where do you feel is the safest place to give birth and why? (hospital/birthing center/home)

 ____

 ____

7. List two healthy habits you plan to adopt now that you are pregnant.

 a. ____

 b. ____

8. How much exercise do you get and which type do you think is healthy during pregnancy?

 ____

 ____

9. Name one thing you would like from others that would help you with this pregnancy.

 ____

 ____

10. List three things you do to pamper yourself on a monthly basis.

 a. ____

 b. ____

 c. ____

I hope this exercise has helped you increase awareness of how you feel about your pregnancy, and helps you realize whether you need to do something differently. If on question 10, you answered, "get a massage," stop and make an appointment even if it is with your partner. If you answered, "eating at a favorite restaurant," make reservations. Do it because you deserve it. You are carrying the baby.

So, What's Next?

Your first response may be that these questions were easy and fun. While you may have already thought about the changes that pregnancy will bring, you will find that writing down your thoughts may stimulate new meaning. You may have experienced some fears or negative feelings, causing you to become apprehensive; addressing the reasons behind some of these fears or negative feelings can be scary but also very empowering.

Special Note:

I want to take this time to make all readers aware that I know from my experience as a nurse practitioner, lactation consultant, Lamaze instructor, and birth/postpartum doula that many women have experienced trauma in their lives. If the above questionnaire made you feel nervous or afraid of your upcoming birth, please discuss this with your healthcare provider. Some of you may have experienced trauma during your childhood, like physical, emotional or sexual abuse. This pregnancy and birth can bring issues to the surface causing you to experience anxiety or panic attacks. Some issues can cause you to feel uncomfortable, while others can produce painful memories. Dealing with these painful issues by talking with your healthcare provider or by finding a counselor who specializes in helping abuse survivors may help you cope with your feelings. This can be a difficult subject to discuss. You are not alone. This may be a family secret and the information you share with your midwife, doctor or counselor will be kept private.

Developing the "I can handle it" Attitude

So, how do you take this information about your beliefs of pregnancy to create the pregnancy and birth the way you wish? Start with positive thinking. You can develop confidence in your body and yourself by developing the "I can handle it" attitude. Start now. Say these four words aloud: "I can handle it." Again: "I can handle it." By developing this "I can handle it" attitude, your confidence level increases and you will realize you have the ability and thought processes to handle anything that comes your way. You may presently be experiencing morning sickness, and even though it's not fun, it will pass and you can handle it. Or you may be dealing with more serious medical issues like gestational diabetes or pregnancy induced hypertension; keep saying to yourself, "I can handle it," and then examine the options.

Getting Yourself to the Next Level of Belief

I plan to show you techniques to enhance your joy, to build confidence, to help decrease your stress and eliminate many of your fears and concerns in regards to pregnancy, birth and parenthood. As you read and understand these techniques, you will need to practice them daily until you have mastered them. You will see your life begin to open up in ways you never thought possible. When you see these positive changes, you will want to continue using these techniques in every facet of your life, through pregnancy and beyond.

Positive Thinking

Much has been written in recent years about the importance of positive thinking and the belief that life is abundant. Not only do I believe in positive thinking and life's abundance, I personally use the techniques I will teach you and have seen changes in my life.

One thing that held me back, and that holds most people back, is a negative mindset, which is developed by what we have always heard (daily conversations), what we were taught (parent's belief, friends, school, newspapers, books, etc.), and what we have opened our minds to accept. Most people are their own worst enemy, just by the sheer fact of the negative daily conversations they have with themselves. This self-talk can be so familiar, you may not be aware of this destructive behavior. You have convinced yourself of things that may not have any truth to them at all. Some people are more negative than others. Try to go all week without saying a negative comment or without criticizing someone or something. We get into a habit of negative comments and soon this becomes our normal conversation with ourselves.

Let me give you an example of negative self-talk in regards to pregnancy:

> "I can't believe I'm pregnant, I am going to get so fat and won't be able to wear any of my skinny jeans, I can't believe my doctor expects me to get on the scale every visit and embarrass me about the 'big number.' I know my coworkers can see how bad my skin is breaking out; I know this baby is going to take all my spare time and I won't get to be with my friends ever again, my doctor didn't talk much at my appointment today… I know she thinks I gained too much weight or maybe she doesn't like me. I wanted to talk about my birth plan, but I know she'll think it's stupid and I don't want to upset her.
>
> "My partner didn't kiss me last night… he thinks I'm unattractive, and isn't as happy about the baby as I am... I know by the way he's acting… his mother asked about my last doctor's appointment… I know she just wants to know all my private medical history…"

STOP! STOP! STOP!
STOP THE NEGATIVE TALK!

Can you see how this negative talk continues to grow? How do you stop it? Here's your first step to change or to embrace the way you see life…be prepared to be amazed. Starting now, it's time for you to change the way you talk to yourself. One of the easiest and quickest ways to turn your negative thinking around is to start with positive self-talk.

In the blank journal pages at the back of this book, you'll find space to write your positive affirmations. Here is an example of five positive affirmations:

1. I am a strong woman.
2. I can trust my body.
3. I am sending positive energy to my baby.
4. I am eating healthily for my baby.
5. I am a happy person.

Now, I suggest you copy these in the blank journal pages in the back of this book. Then, add five more statements. They must start with "I am / will / can..."

If you are the partner, your affirmations should read like this:

1. I am a good provider.
2. I am successful.
3. I am a kind and understanding person.
4. I am proud of my partner and baby.
5. I am excited about being a parent.

Add five more statements to your list.

After writing at least ten positive affirmations, you will now stand tall, with shoulders back, in front of a mirror and state aloud your list of positive statements. This part feels silly but is a must in order for your brain to process this change. Do this twice a day—once in the morning and once before retiring to bed. Look at yourself as you repeat each statement. Marshall Sylver's book *Passion, Profit and Power* presents studies that show it takes twenty-one days of repeating an act before it becomes a habit. Even after twenty-one days, I believe we need to work every day on keeping our thinking in the direction that serves us the best.

Another way to change the negative thinking is to post positive quotes all around the house, at your office, in the car, on the fridge, in the bathroom, or on your computer screen.

Here are a few of my favorites:

- "Life isn't about how to survive the storm, but how to dance in the rain." —Author unknown
- "A mind once expanded can never contract to its original size." —Ralph Waldo Emerson
- "Don't ask for fewer problems, ask for more wisdom." —Jim Rohm
- "In communication you get back what you send out." —Marshall Sylver

Heighten Your Awareness

You're changing your thinking by using positive affirmations and by posting your favorite quotes in your room, car and office. Now it's time to heighten your awareness of nature and all things that grow and bloom without effort. John Gray, a leading expert on relationships and author of the *Men are from Mars, Women are from Venus* book series, states in the video *New Beginnings - Pregnancy, Partnership and Participation* that the pregnant woman must get in tune with nature, strengthen her faith in God, or her faith in Mother Nature. Once, the culture surrounding women was very different. Woman's role as mother, life-giver, and nurturer was celebrated and held sacred. Pregnant women were seen as very special. Today, although we think a pregnant woman is special, we nevertheless expect her to continue to work her job, take care of the home, and take on activities outside the house. A pregnant woman needs to take on less. She needs to learn how to say no. She needs to take time to "stop and smell the roses." She needs to become aware of her body's signals, to rest when she is tired, to drink when she is thirsty, and to eat what her body needs.

In order to do these things, you need to cultivate sensory awareness. This next exercise will help you do this. On a beautiful day as you walk at your favorite park, when you stop and observe nature, all of your senses will be heightened.

Sensory Awareness Exercise

On your 30-minute walk, notice nature around you. Observe how the trees and flowers bloom with the season, how grass grows with the right nutrients, including water and sun. Notice the time of day—where's the sun or moon? Notice the temperature and smells of the air, the different textures of nature.

During this walk, you may think about your own childhood and the good memories you want your child to also have; like playing in the back yard on the swing set, climbing trees, riding bikes, coloring a beautiful picture for your mother or father, playing with baby dolls, tea parties, dress up, having a supportive family and learning many life lessons while knowing you felt secure and loved. Remember that all good thoughts bring a surge of endorphins, which send a positive feeling to your baby. You can increase this surge by receiving a tender kiss or comforting hug from your partner.

Practice this exercise every opportunity you can. The more often you visualize a positive image, the clearer your vision becomes. If your childhood was not pleasant, kind or loving, it is very important that you get counseling and figure out what you want for your baby. If you don't have a positive vision, learned negative behaviors from your past will continue. In the meantime, make believe "as if"... as if you already have everything you dreamed... a caring relationship, peace in your life, owning a home, supportive family, successful career, etc.

Each time you do a sensory awareness walk in nature, you will notice more examples of simple beauty, develop a sense of peace and just be plain amazed. These nature adventures will become part of your routine.

As you walk, start thinking about your healthcare provider: Why did you choose this midwife or doctor? Do you feel comfortable asking her questions? Does she support your wishes for birth? If you are shy about asking questions, start practicing by asking her questions aloud while you walk. By doing this, you will become comfortable with starting conversations with your midwife or doctor and be able to ask pertinent questions.

Relaxation Techniques

Another way to increase self-awareness, and an important part of an easier and shorter labor, is to use the art of relaxation. You will need to practice this daily, especially during the last four weeks. These techniques are good for life, not just for labor.

Progressive Relaxation

As you find a comfortable place, give yourself permission to relax for the next twenty minutes. Sit in a comfortable chair that supports your arms and head or lie down in bed. Take a deep breath, in through your nose out through your mouth… now take another deep breath and this time as you exhale, make a sigh sound… that's it... relax all your muscles… let go… allow your muscles to become loose, limp and relaxed.

If you have had a stressful day, visualize taking all your unfinished work, unanswered phone calls, or incomplete chores and put them in a small box. Once you put the top on this box, you will not think about this box until your relaxation session is completed. If your mind wanders, gently draw your attention back to the rhythm of your breathing.

Start with your feet… move your feet around, relaxing all the tiny muscles on the tops of your feet as well as on the bottoms. Fan your toes apart… that's it… a nice stretch… rest your feet in a comfortable position… let this relaxation move up your calves and thighs… you can relax one leg at a time or both at the same time. Take a deep breath, and as you inhale, slightly squeeze your legs together or if you're on your back, press your legs against the bed or chair… as you exhale, relax… let your muscles become loose, limp and relaxed.

Let this relaxation move into your pelvis. Take a deep breath… relax your pelvic muscle, the muscle that you tighten when you stop the flow of urine… breathe in… slightly tighten the muscles of your pelvis… exhale… relax… that's it… now, relax your buttock muscles… you may need to shift your bottom in order to get this group of muscles loose and let go…

Breathe deeply… inhale, and relax as you exhale… relax your abdominal muscles, allow your tummy to sag… relax the muscles across your chest… big breath in and big breath out.

As you inhale, slowly stretch your arms down by your side toward your knees, a nice stretch… now exhale and relax your arms… fan open your hands… stretching your fingers… that's it, stretch… now relax… inhale… exhale… relax… loose, limp and relaxed.

Next, you will be relaxing your back… since this is a large area, we will divide it into the upper and lower halves… concentrate on the lower half of your back… visualize the air you're breathing warming up as it passes through your nose or mouth, down your throat and into your lungs... this air continues to get warmer… visualize that your lungs are like ovens… as the air enters, it heats up… Now, visualize exhaling this hot air through small pores in your back. As this hot air warms your muscles, you relax… that's it... relax those tiny muscles in your lower back… as your muscles feel this warmth they relax and let go… now repeat this breathing of air… visualize your breath as it goes down your throat, warmer… warmer… into the lungs… and exhale your hot breath through the small pores in your back between your shoulder blades… think of a heating pad or warm water on your back. That's it… relax… inhale… relax as you exhale.

Relax your shoulders… shrug your shoulders up toward your ears as you inhale… hold them there… now relax as you exhale… your muscles should be loose, limp and relaxed.

Next you will relax your neck... inhale, and slowly stretch your chin toward your chest... bring your head back to its normal position, then slowly stretch toward one shoulder, then the other... You may need to stretch several times in order to relax your neck muscles… exhale and relax.

Move this relaxation over your scalp and across your face. Your eyelids still feel very heavy… your cheeks feel like they are drooping… drop your lower jaw… move it from side to side… relax your tongue so that it fills the entire cavity of your mouth.

Now your entire body should be relaxed… focus on your breathing… notice how your chest slowly rises and falls… each time you take a breath, say to yourself as you inhale… "I am" and as you exhale, say "relaxed"… repeat this five times… inhale, "I am"…exhale, "relaxed"… inhale, "I am"…exhale, "relaxed"... Each time you repeat these three words, you become more relaxed.

If you are listening to music, close your eyes and allow your mind to focus on that for the next few minutes, keeping your body in this heightened relaxed state. When you are ready, take a deep breath, stretch your arms and legs…that's it… just enjoy for a moment longer… when you open your eyes you will feel full of energy and ready to go.

One good way to enhance your relaxation is by adding visualization. I have written three different scripts; please feel free to create your own. Many mothers have their partners describe the details of one of their favorite vacation trips.

I have alternated the usage of "him" and "her" pronouns in the visualization scripts for easier reading and to make the visualizations more personal. Please substitute the gender of your baby (if you know it), or whichever gender you wish when you read or listen to your recording of the visualization.

Baby's Nursery

Visualize that you are sitting in a comfortable rocking chair in your baby's completed nursery…you begin to rock back and forth…back and forth…it's been a hectic last five days since the birth of your child… this is the first quiet moment you have had with your baby… see your baby in your arms…your baby is awake, alert, staring into your face… you are gazing into your baby's eyes… love is being shared…take this time to notice the tiny features of your baby's face…notice your baby's hair... what color is it? How much does she have? Is it curly or straight? Look at the shape and color of your baby's eyes, notice the eyebrows and eyelashes, the shape of your baby's nose, the delicate lips…Look closely at the fine, downy hair (lanugo) that covers your baby's face… Notice the shape of your baby's ears... Your baby is still gazing into your face, studying your face looking intently at all of your features… Put your finger in the palm of her hand… as she tries to close her hand around your finger, notice the tiny, perfectly shaped nails and the creases at each joint… You smile with wonder, amazement, and the true feeling of love, and she smiles back at you.

As you continue to rock back and forth, while talking with your baby, make a promise to this baby as to what type of parent you plan to be…next, tell your baby one thing you will do for her… Tell her one thing from your childhood that was exciting and/or meaningful that you wish for her… think of one place you would like to take your child when she gets older…tell her one wonderful trait your partner has that you hope she has… As she drifts off to sleep in your arms, tell her you will love her for always…love her forever.

Now, return to your present place. The day will come when you will have many hours of quiet rocking and conversations with your child… Cherish each one… Take a deep breath…when you open your eyes, you will be filled with energy.

Trip to the Beach

Imagine that you are sitting in a comfortable chair on your favorite beach. This chair has a high back to rest your head and wide armrest so there's plenty of room for your arms to be completely supported. Move your feet around in the sand… feel the warmth... feel the smoothness of the sand as it goes between your toes… now rest your feet and legs in a comfortable position.

Look out at the ocean… notice the size of the waves… are there any white caps, or is it a calm day? How does the water look? Is it gray or blue or deep green? Listen to the sound of the waves as they hit the beach… are they softly lapping, or are they louder, crashing on the shoreline? Feel the energy from the massive body of water… feel the power. As you sit with palms facing up, relaxed on the arms of the chair… visualize all negativity leaving through your feet into the earth... all fear, stress, worry, anger, doubt, draining into the sand and to the sea to be carried away... When completely empty of negative energy, allow the surging, powerful, positive energy of the ocean to enter your body through your fingertips, filling your whole body with positive energy… giving you power. Notice the movement of this energy; sometimes you will imagine it moving slow and other times, more quickly. Visualize it moving up your arms and down through your chest, filling your chest and abdomen, continuing its path to your pelvis, moving downward, filling your thighs, calves, each of your feet and every toe. Even with your body energized, you can continue to feel relaxed… take a deep breath... in through your nose or mouth and with a soft sigh, exhale… relax all your muscles.

Your awareness of all your senses has been heightened… hear the movement of water as it comes in and goes out… smell the air, salty, fresh… Feel the warm breeze as it crosses your body. All the nerve endings on your skin are stimulated, it feels good, and you also notice that as soon as your skin is getting a little warm, another breeze blows in softly... cooling and soothing… Let your mind wander... picture your favorite day at the beach… Who was with you…What did you enjoy? As you think about this wonderful time in your life, relax all your muscles, take several deep breaths, and enjoy this vision.

With your eyes still closed, your body relaxed, visualize your little three-year-old child playing in the sand just a few feet in front of you. He is making sandcastles and talking to himself, using his imagination… A big smile shines on his face, amazed at his ability to flip the bucketful of sand and make a perfect sand castle. You are so in love with him… you never could have imagined loving someone so much. Each day he brings joy to your life and at the end of the day as you tuck him in, you will sigh as a sense of peace and calm fills the room. Your active child is asleep. You smile as you gaze down at his sweet, angelic face. This child is a gift that you have been given. You will provide love and guidance. You will nurture, teach life lessons to and cherish this gift. Life is precious…so many people take it for granted…you will not take any day for granted.

Return to your present place…take a deep breath… feel the ocean's breeze moving across your skin and the energy that fills your body. Take another deep breath, bringing more oxygen to all your muscles and cells. You will have a wonderful day or night. You will have stored energy for whenever you need it. Slowly open your eyes while you inhale… stretch… exhale…

You are ready to go.

Autumn Walk

Today, you have decided to take a visit to the mountains. Visualize yourself driving up into the mountains. You anticipate the beautiful fall colors. As you get closer to the top of the mountain, you park your car, stand at the lookout spot and gaze out at the beauty. The colors of the leaves are more vibrant than you had imagined. You notice a path leading into the woods… it's a path that has been walked many times before... notice how the leaves are packed down into a smooth brown walkway, making your entrance into the woods easy... As you enter, everything appears still and quiet... Walking a bit further, you see a huge, old oak tree surrounded by a large, light green, thick carpet of moss.

You sit and rest your back against the trunk of this mighty oak... the carpet of moss cushions your buttocks... take a deep breath... relax your entire body... another deep breath... as you exhale, gaze up toward the sky... Notice the sun peaking through the trees...the bright light reflects against the colorful leaves... Notice the red ones... the yellow ones... the orange ones... the green ones... Take a deep breath... inhale slowly... exhale... relax. As your body and mind become relaxed and quiet, your senses become more tuned in to your surroundings...

The sun is rather hot but the shade from the trees keeps the heat off your body... The soft green moss is cooling your body. Close your eyes and listen... hear the leaves moving with the gentle breeze... relax your body even more... hear birds singing in the distance... deeper relaxation... hear squirrels playing and chasing each other from tree to tree.

You are so relaxed, you find yourself drifting off to sleep... After a few minutes, you think you hear water trickling over rocks... for a moment you are in such a dream state you can't tell if it's real or make-believe... continue to listen quietly... after 30 seconds or so, you feel you must open your eyes...

When you open your eyes, you glance over your right shoulder and, to your surprise, you notice a small brook with a stream of clear water bubbling over smooth stones... a young fawn and its mother are drinking from this brook. You look up into the trees, noticing again the colors of the leaves... yellow ones, orange ones, red ones, and green ones... You see two squirrels playing and jumping from tree to tree... notice the bright red cardinal, look at his deep red feathers gleaming alongside the vibrancy of the leaves on the maple tree in front of you.

Time has slipped away, and the sun is beginning to set. The air is noticeably cooler... the forest is becoming quiet for the day...the squirrels have stopped playing... the singing of the birds grows quieter, calmer... Take a deep breath and continue to relax for a minute longer... You stand from your carpet of soft moss and begin walking back toward the small path where you started... You reach the edge of the woods, look back and imprint in your mind the memories of today... Remember the smoothness of the brown leaves, the snapping of the twigs under your feet as you walked down the path, the coolness of the air as the sun begins to set, the calmness of the forest... Look one more time at the beauty of the changing leaves... the yellow ones, orange ones, red ones, green ones... these colors are truly nature's gift of the changing season.

Take a deep breath... return to this room... stretch, and your next deep breath will fill you with plenty of energy. Open your eyes. Big breath... Enjoy your day.

When you find yourself returning to this vision, you can also reflect about the changes in life that are beautiful: falling in love, creating life, growing your baby, giving birth, supporting your partner, sharing with your baby your gifts and talents, teaching your child life lessons and always remembering that being the parent of this child is a privilege. Children are the gifts in life. They give unconditional love, which teaches us lessons about patience and persistence. They will also spend your money and pluck your last nerve while giving more hours of laughter than you can imagine!

Remember:

- Your mindset of pregnancy—begin to understand your belief systems and develop a positive picture.
- Develop the "I can handle it" attitude.
- Start believing in yourself by trusting your body and trusting your baby.
- Relaxation is the key to bring a calm, peaceful state to your mind and body, not just for pregnancy but also for life.
- Enjoy your self-awareness nature walks.

CHAPTER TWO

Your Birth Plan

As the weeks pass, your baby and your excitement continue to grow. The much anticipated event of the birth will soon be a reality. During this part of your journey of discovery, you will examine your fears and share an emotional and spiritual bonding with your partner as you build self-confidence by learning to trust your body.

Before you can accomplish all this, there are several things you need to do. You should take stock of your current mindset on birth, and create a birth plan. Take a few minutes to address the prompts and questions listed below, using the supplemental section of blank journal pages in the back of this book. After completing these "Your Mindset for Birth" questions, you may notice many of your answers are based on your subconscious thinking. I will explain more about how our subconscious thinking affects our every day decisions, and how planning ahead by creating a birth plan can help to create more desirable outcomes.

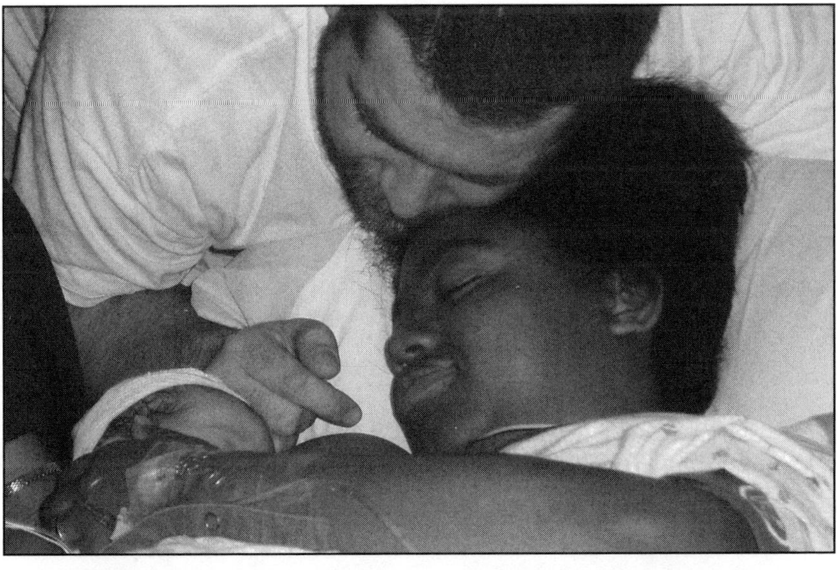

Candace and Hunter bonding with their daughter, Phoenix.

Your Mindset for Birth

1. List three things you believe would make your birth experience meaningful.

   a. Stafford very involved

   b. To be aware + able to move

   c. Hold baby immediately

2. List any fears or concerns you wish your healthcare provider to know.

   Not having birth plan supported, Not being informed ab interventions or what is happening to my body/er baby

3. Think of three actions/techniques that you use now to get into a relaxed state.

   a. deep breathing

   b. Showers

   c. yoga/meditation + mantras

4. Write two things that you want your partner to know/remember in order to support you during birth.

   a. Advocate for our plan for me+baby

   b. Have faith that I can do this + remind me

5. Where do you think is the safest place for you to give birth and why?

   Hospital, in case anything goes wrong

6. Who do you wish to be present during labor (partner, doula, doctor / midwife / family)?

Stafford, midwife, doctor if needed

7. Do you trust your body's ability to birth your baby? If yes, what are your strengths? If no, why not?

yes, I am determined, ive challenged my body physically before

8. Write one memory of what members of your family (grandmother / mother / sister / aunts) always talked about in regards to birth.

9. If there were absolutely no medical or safety issues for you or your baby, what might be your "fantasy birth"? Include anything you would love to experience during your birth such as a water birth, birthing in the warm ocean or a lagoon, birthing at home in your own quiet bedroom with your midwife and family, birthing in a beautiful garden surrounded by nature, etc.

Hopefully, these questions have helped you look more closely at your current thinking on birth. Now I would like for you to decide whether your responses are based on truth or on myth. Maybe your subconscious thinking is holding you back. Maybe what holds you back is a lack of knowledge and understanding. Or maybe you have read and educated yourself, and you are happy and comfortable with all your beliefs about giving birth. When you are comfortable with your birth options, you will be able to relax and enjoy your birth experience. If you still feel unsettled or uneasy about any of your decisions, examining your feelings and changing your current thinking, or coming to terms with it, can bring peace to your mind, allowing you to trust your body as well as the decisions about your birth plan.

So, what is subconscious thinking and how can one change it? Many of our actions are based on thoughts and suppositions that we have told ourselves are true, whether they are or not. Over time, such thoughts can become ingrained in the subconscious mind, and form our beliefs about life, ourselves and others. These beliefs cause us to decide what things are true or untrue, good or bad, and right or wrong for ourselves and for those we love.

As a young child, your belief system is usually the same as that of your parents. You are also influenced by your own experiences and forces in the outside world, such as extended family, friends, teachers, television, internet, magazines, billboards, etc. Much of our belief system is strongly present by the time we reach age eight. We believe the things that we have been taught and what we think we know are the truth, despite the fact that some, or even all, of the information fed to us may be incorrect. All the decisions we make are based on these supposed truths. According to Marshall Sylver, author of *Passion, Profit, and Power*, "every action you do either is consciously or unconsciously motivated by a thought. This thought is the cause; the action we take is the effect. To change the action, we first need to change the thought."

How Do You Change Your Subconscious Mind?

First, you need to become aware of your current mindset. Then, you need to crystallize your own vision of your goal. What do you want? If you find that your current mindset is blocking you from achieving your goal, then you need to start reprogramming your thinking—changing your subconscious mind.

One of the ways you can begin to reprogram your thinking is by changing your daily self-talk. Using positive affirmations like, "It is easy for me to change," or, "I will achieve my goal of ______________________ with grace and ease," can help you to do this. If one of your goals is to have a low intervention birth, you need to program your thinking to achieve this goal. Use daily self-talk affirmations such as, "It will be easy for me to relax during labor even if contractions are strong and uncomfortable," and, "I can trust my body. It knows what to do." Here is a great quote by Mike Dooley, author of *Infinite Possibilities,* that is worth remembering: "Thoughts become things. Choose the good ones."

How do you presently visualize your upcoming birth? Until you become aware of your present mindset about birth, you don't know whether you need to change any of your current thoughts or actions. After completing the "Your Mindset for Birth" questions, clear your mind of any fears or obstacles and in the blank journal pages in the back of this book, begin to write your ideal birth. In your ideal birth, there is no need to worry about or to include any hint of safety or medical concerns. Your ideal birth is completely safe, resulting in a healthy baby and mother, whatever details you include, whatever the setting happens to be. Be creative. Go wild! As you begin to think about your ideal birth, consider the following things:

Where would you like to have your baby? At home, in a birthing center, a hospital? Describe your surroundings.

What type of support do you wish to receive? Continuous support from your husband, partner, mother, sister, friend or a hired birth doula, or some other kind of support person?

Do you want to have low intervention or do you plan to get an epidural as soon as you get to the hospital?

Who is going to provide you with medical care—a midwife or a doctor?

Have you written or thought of a birth plan?

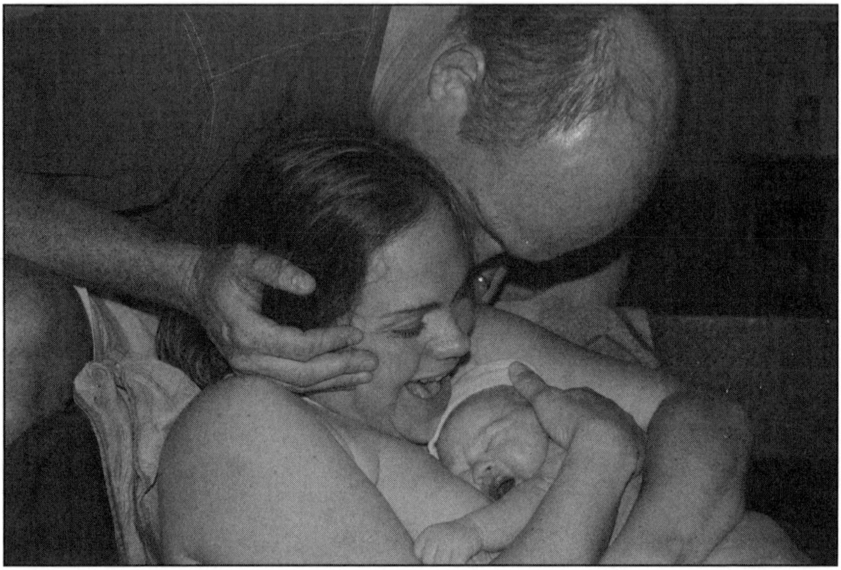

Sandra and Bruce chose a homebirth for the birth of their second son.

When you are finished, you may find that you have written a very safe, comfortable vision of your ideal birth. But what if, secretly, you would really like to give birth in water, or you've considered low intervention birth but are afraid to say so for fear of failure? Write it down and make it happen. Your personal desires and wishes can be honored if you would only ask. Ask and you may receive it all. If you never ask, you will never know. The birth plan becomes an important communication tool between mother and partner, mother and healthcare provider, mother and hospital staff. It contains a written collection of your desires in order to make this birth meaningful as you welcome your baby into his new world.

Writing Your Birth Plan

You may decide to include many of the following items in your birth plan. Write your birth plan in an order that works for you. It may be in a checklist format or a written prose format.

Full Circle Childbirth Consultants, Inc.
Birth Plan

Mother's Name ____________ **Support Person** ____________

Doctor ____________ **Due Date** ____________

First Stage

Positions
- Walking ____
- Standing ____
- Rocking ____
- Lunge ____
- Sitting ____
- Birth Ball ____
- Lying Down ____
- Back of Bed ____

Comfort Measures
- Showers ____
- Massage ____
- Hot Packs ____
- Cold Packs ____
- Music ____

Phone
- Incoming calls ____
- Only call out ____

Fluids
- Ice Chips ____
- Ice Pops ____
- Juice ____
- I.V. ____

Monitor
- Continuous ____
- Intermittent ____
- External ____
- Internal ____

Medication
- None ____
- Narcotics ____
- Epidural ____

Second Stage

Positions
- Squatting ____
- Side Lying ____
- Semi Sitting ____
- Hands & Knees ____

Perineal Care
- Perineal Massage ____
- Warm Compresses ____
- Episiotomy ____

Positions you would like to use for the first phase of labor:

- Walking
- Standing
- Rocking
- Using a birth ball
- Sitting
- Lying Down
- Leaning over the back of the bed—especially helpful for back labor

Comfort measures you may want during your labor:

- Shower or tub
- Massage
- Essential oil blends for calming and nausea
- Hot Packs
- Cold Packs
- Wearing your own clothes
- Music

Fluids you would like access to:

- Ice Chips
- Ice Pops
- Juice
- Herbal teas—raspberry leaf tea
- IV—intravenous fluids
- Heparin/saline lock

Preferences for types of fetal monitoring:

- Continuous: monitoring fetus during entire labor (See Chapter 3 for a description of this procedure.)
- Intermittent: monitoring fetus 10 to 20 minutes of every hour then off to move freely in room or hallway
- External: belts around the belly that holds monitor in place
- Internal: monitor that is inserted into baby's scalp

Preferences regarding medication(s):

- None

- Narcotics, pain medications
- Epidural (See Chapter 3 for a description of this procedure.)

Positions you might wish to use during second stage of labor:
- Squatting
- Side-lying
- Semi-sitting
- Hands and knees

Wishes for immediate postpartum care in hospital:
- Keeping your baby on your chest during the initial exam
- Father or partner to cut the umbilical cord
- Breastfeeding during the first 30 minutes
- Rooming in—partial or total. You can request that your baby stay in the room with you throughout your hospital stay or that she sleep in the nursery for as much time as is comfortable for you.
- Visitors limited or not
- Delay eye care. As a matter of course, hospitals generally apply antibiotic ointment to a baby's eyes after birth to guard against any infection that may be transmitted from mother to baby through the trip down the birth canal. If there is no danger of infection, you may request that eye care be delayed.
- Discuss vaccines with your pediatrician
- Do you wish to give your baby his first bath?
- Would you like pictures taken during labor and delivery?

These are just a few suggestions to think about when writing your birth plan. Consider for yourself what's important for you. Many of these items will be discussed in your childbirth preparation class. It is very important to communicate with your healthcare provider and doula any major fears or concerns. Many people fear needles. Many people fear the very idea of pain, or of losing control. By discussing these concerns, you can discover options to decrease your fears.

Your birth plan will help communicate to the nursing staff your desires. Some nurses will be willing to work with your birth plan. Others are not as receptive and you may find yourself having to negotiate all your wishes while dealing with labor. This is another good reason to have your birth plan blessed by your healthcare provider. Your partner also needs to be your advocate, along with your birth doula. Nurses may be busy with other patients, leaving little extra time to offer to you. Touring the hospital before birth will also give you an idea of the attitude of the nurses that work in labor and delivery. Changing hospitals is sometimes an option, and for those of you who don't have that option, talk with the head nurse of the labor and delivery unit. Express your concerns and desires. Ask her for help to make this birth experience the most memorable for you and your partner. If you get a nurse that just doesn't click, ask for a new nurse, one who likes to work with low intervention births.

Be sure to remember that your birth plan needs to be flexible, meaning that if you or your baby's health is in immediate need of emergency care, all or most of your personal requests may be tabled. Most couples know this and absolutely want only the best for both mother and baby.

I have included samples of birth plans in the appendices of this book. You may also find samples of birth plans on internet sites such as www.Babycenter.com or www.birthplan.com. Both sites demonstrate birth plans with similar formats, and will ask you to include the following information: your name, your support person(s) name, including your doula, clothes you wish to wear during labor, preferred comfort measures and positions for labor, such as walking, standing, using the birth ball, laboring in the shower or tub, and interventions, like intermittent vs. continuous fetal monitoring, internal or external fetal monitoring, IV fluids or ice pops and juices, your wishes regarding medications, episiotomy, perineal massage, and a variety of positions you might prefer for pushing your baby out.

The most important part of the birth plan is that it gives you the opportunity to write down your wishes, concerns, fears, and desires. This information allows your healthcare provider and nursing staff to provide more specialized care, and it gives you a greater sense of control.

You may find that many of your concerns and fears can be addressed early on, even months before the birth. If you fear the pain of birth in general, or if you have a fear of what you believe an intervention procedure will be, like the fear of needles for an IV or an epidural, you must understand that the fear itself can cause intense physical tension. Your body will respond to this tension by prolonging your labor. Educate yourself by asking questions of your healthcare provider, and by attending childbirth classes or mother support groups. Realize that learning about specific interventions can help you alleviate these fears as well as help you to trust your body and your instincts. Your body is capable of knowing which hormones to produce when it's time for labor to begin and to produce uterine contractions that allow your cervix to dilate and efface (open and thin). Your body also responds positively to a calm, quiet and relaxed state. Trust your body.

What happens when you can't relax or if you become very stressed due to the unfamiliar environment or the discomfort and pain of labor? When a woman becomes stressed, or is frightened, her body is programmed to produce stress hormones known as catecholamines. These hormones automatically trigger her to respond with the fight or flight response. When these hormones are dumped into the bloodstream during the first stage of labor, the body responds by decreasing blood flow to the uterus and decreasing uterine contractions. This will inevitably increase the duration of the first stage of labor. When a birthing woman's body is triggered to respond as though there is a threat to either her safety, or that of her baby, blood flow to the placenta is decreased, causing not only the mother, but the fetus, to produce catecholamines, as well as the accompanying bodily responses, including increased heart rate and blood pressure. Over a long period of time, this continued stress can cause fetal distress.

Stress, Pain, and Catecholamines

by Penny Simkin, PT, CD (DONA) 2002

Maternal Effects of Anxiety ("Tend and Befriend" response) in Labor

Excessive catecholamine levels in first stage of labor→

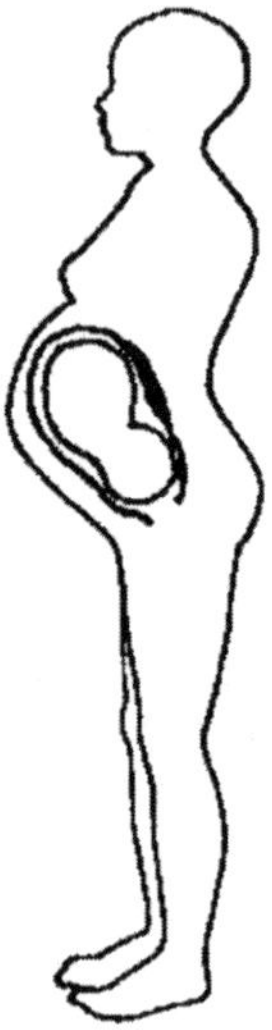

↓ blood flow to uterus

↓ uterine contractions

↑ duration of first stage of labor

↓ blood flow to placenta

↑ fetal production of catecholamines

- Fetal conservation of oxygen
- Fetal heart rate decelerations

↑ negative or pessimistic perception of events by woman

↑ need for reassurance & support

Excessive catecholamine levels in second stage labor →

- Same fetal effects as listed above
- "fetal ejection reflex" (rapid expulsion of fetus)

The woman benefits from avoidance or reduction of stress.

Permission granted by Penny Simkin to use this diagram.

Knowing that this kind of hormonal stress response exists should give you good reason to want to practice relaxation techniques. You need to become aware of any environmental, as well as personal, stressors that may trigger stress for you. Learn your stressors; listen to your body, rest when you need to rest, eat when you are hungry while you are at home in labor, relax when your uterus is contracting. Learn to move your body both for comfort and in order to best utilize gravity to help move your baby down the birth canal, and before long she will be in your arms, looking in your eyes and this new love affair will change your world.

Think for a moment about your baby's first minutes, about what it must be like arriving into a strange, cold, brightly lit room, not knowing where she is or what is happening, or why she has been removed from the warm, comforting environment that has been her home for so many weeks, and then suddenly finding the comfort of your warm arms, your sweet smell, and your beautiful, welcoming face. Close your eyes and visualize just that moment. After the hard work of labor, as much as your baby is your reward, you are also your baby's.

Typically, couples think about writing a birth plan after attending childbirth education classes, reading a number of pregnancy books, or reviewing internet sites. Many women and couples have usually discussed their birth wishes informally during early pregnancy. As the pregnancy progresses, it becomes pertinent to discuss in greater detail your desires and wishes during birth. You may find that once you and your partner have written out your wishes and desires for labor and birth, your healthcare provider may oppose parts of your plan. Finding yourself at odds with your healthcare provider can put you in a challenging place. Some mothers find that in the beginning, a healthcare provider may verbally support the desire for a low intervention birth, but once her specific wants and needs are put in writing, this healthcare provider's support may change. It is important to negotiate your options with your healthcare provider earlier rather than later. You will need to have this conversation or, if necessary, change to a healthcare provider who will honor your plan before you go into labor. It is better to make a change in your healthcare provider rather than feel that you are not being heard and your wishes are not being respected. This is not an easy decision to make. But you can't relax and labor well if you are angry at your healthcare provider or if you feel that your needs and desires are being dismissed or disregarded. Please note that the hospital where your healthcare provider has privileges may not support some of the items on your birth plan. Hospitals and birthing centers want your business. Talk with the head nurse of labor and delivery or the director of women's services. If mother and baby are healthy and safe, most reasonable requests can be honored.

Doula Support

Have you considered hiring a certified birth doula to provide you and your partner with physical and emotional support during your labor? A doula's support can take a lot of pressure off your partner. With a doula, he doesn't have to remember all the comfort measures, all the breathing and relaxation techniques, while also physically and emotionally supporting you. This may be your first birth and both of you may be unfamiliar with labor and hospital routines. Most doulas will meet with you weeks or even months before your birth and discuss your birth plan. Then she will stay in contact by phone or in person and when you are in labor, she will either come to your home for early labor, or will meet you at the hospital or birthing center, depending on your needs and preferences. She is your advocate, not your voice. She will not perform any medical procedures such as fetal monitoring, taking blood pressure or doing vaginal exams. A doula will make suggestions for different comfort measures

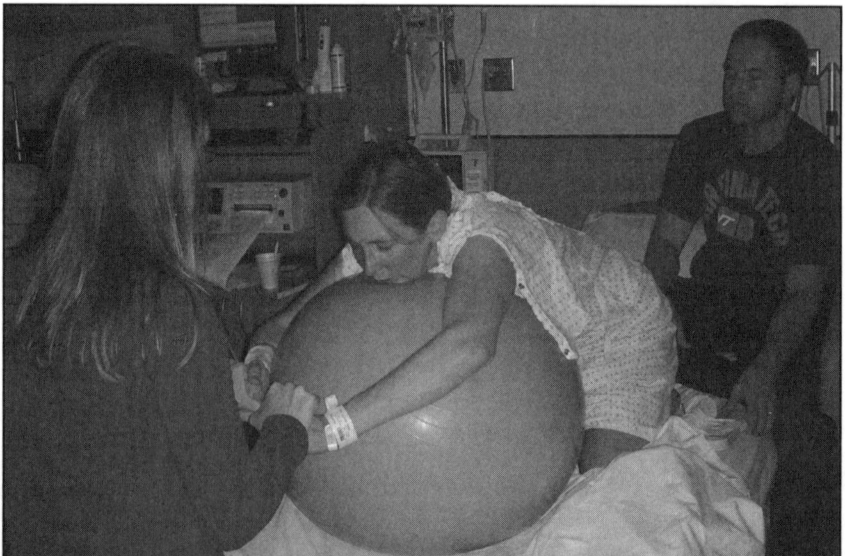

Allison received support from husband, doula and twin sister, Sarah

to aid the mother's relaxation or suggest measures to enhance labor progress and the position of baby. She will be with you throughout your labor and the first hour of postpartum. She will likely visit you and your baby several weeks later to discuss the details of your birth.

Research presented in *Mothering the Mother: How a Doula Can Help You Have a Shorter, Easier and Healthier Birth,* by Marshall H. Klaus, John H. Kennell, and Phyllis H. Klaus (1993), demonstrates that having a doula present at a birth results in the following benefits:

- 50% reduction in the cesarean rate
- 25% shorter labor
- 60% reduction in epidural requests
- 40% reduction in oxytocin use
- 30% reduction in analgesia use
- 40% reduction in forceps delivery

The best way to find a certified doula is to check out the website: DONA.org. You can also find postpartum doulas in your area on this site. Other organizations that certify doulas include CAPPA and LAMAZE. Finding a doula through a professional organization will ensure that the doula you choose has had some formal training and has met certain requirements.

Remember:

- In order to consciously change a belief, you first must picture in your mind what you want.
- Changing your subconscious thinking will require you to use techniques such as positive affirmations, positive self-talk, and listening to relaxation tapes with positive visualizations.
- Reprogramming your subconscious thinking takes 21 days of repetition.
- A written birth plan is a crucial communication tool.
- Hire a certified doula to provide you with physical and emotional support.

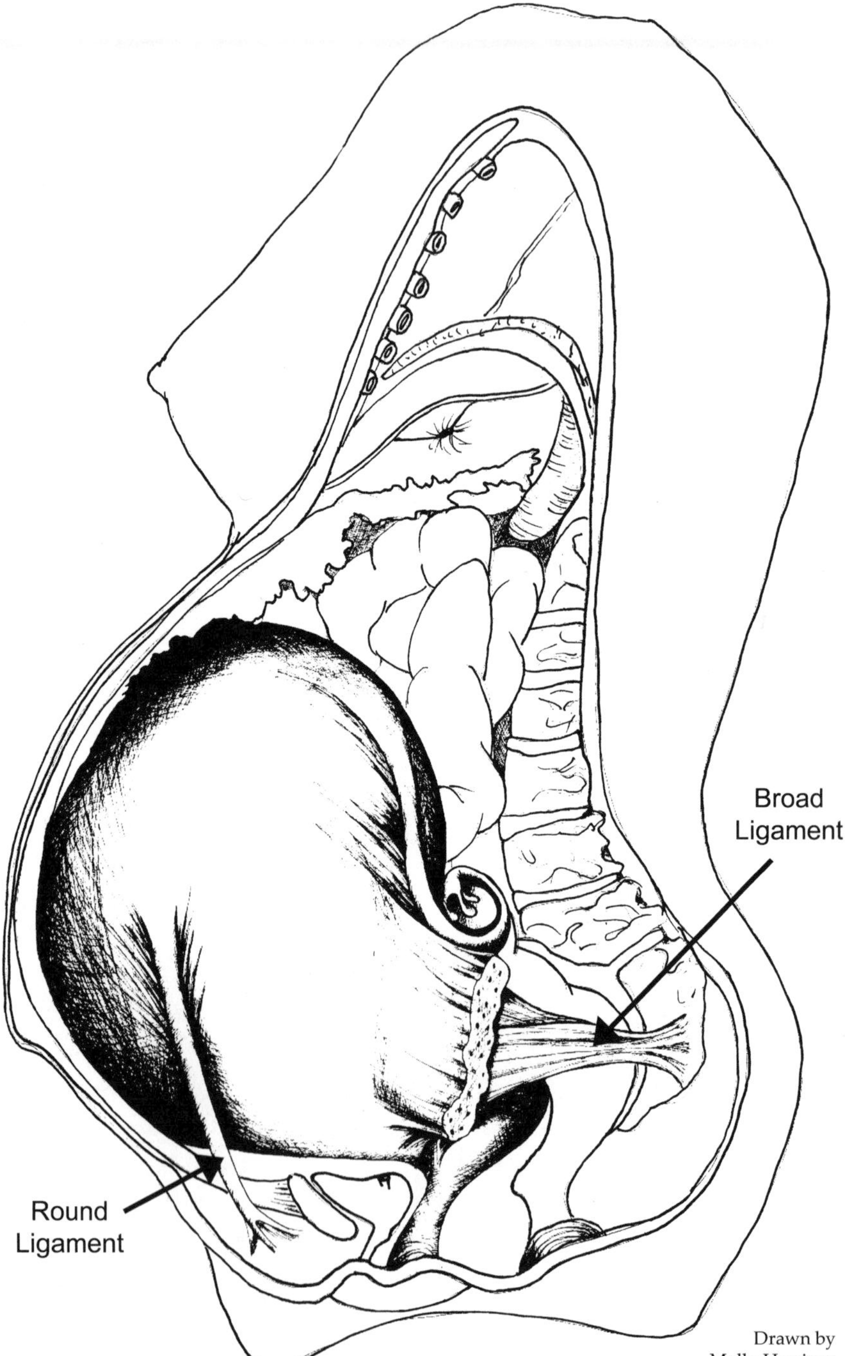
Broad
Ligament
Round
Ligament
Drawn by
Molly Harrison

CHAPTER THREE

Labor and Birth

This chapter will briefly review most topics that are taught in Lamaze-type childbirth class. For greater details and medical research on the use of comfort measures and interventions, I always recommend Penny Simkin's book, *Pregnancy, Childbirth and the Newborn*. Another excellent book to read is *Ina May's Guide to Childbirth* by Ina May Gaskin. A more comprehensive list of childbirth, postpartum, baby care and breastfeeding books can be found in the appendix of this book.

Anatomy and Physiology

The uterus in this diagram describes the position of the round and broad ligaments. The round ligaments are located on each front side in the middle of the uterus and extend downward, attaching to the groin. It supports the uterus as it expands out of the pelvis. During the last few weeks of pregnancy, these ligaments can rapidly contract when you make any sudden moves. It can send a sharp pain down your thigh starting at the groin. When this occurs, flex the affected leg and press three fingers into the groin. You'll find that this pain will ease. If you anticipate any sudden moves like sneezing or coughing, bend or flex your hips.

The broad ligaments attach the uterus to the lower back for support. You may notice aching in your lower back, especially as your belly gets larger and causes strain on those ligaments. Good posture and correct body mechanics can lessen the pain. Having your partner massage this area can feel great and will help you relax and sleep better. You also can help alleviate discomfort by getting on your hands and knees and slowly arching your back upward to the count of five and then returning it to the starting position without sagging. Another technique to aid in relieving this discomfort is to stand with your back against a wall. While standing, press the small of your back flat against the wall…feel the stretch…repeat several times…you should feel less tension on these ligaments.

36 Weeks Gestation Before Lightening

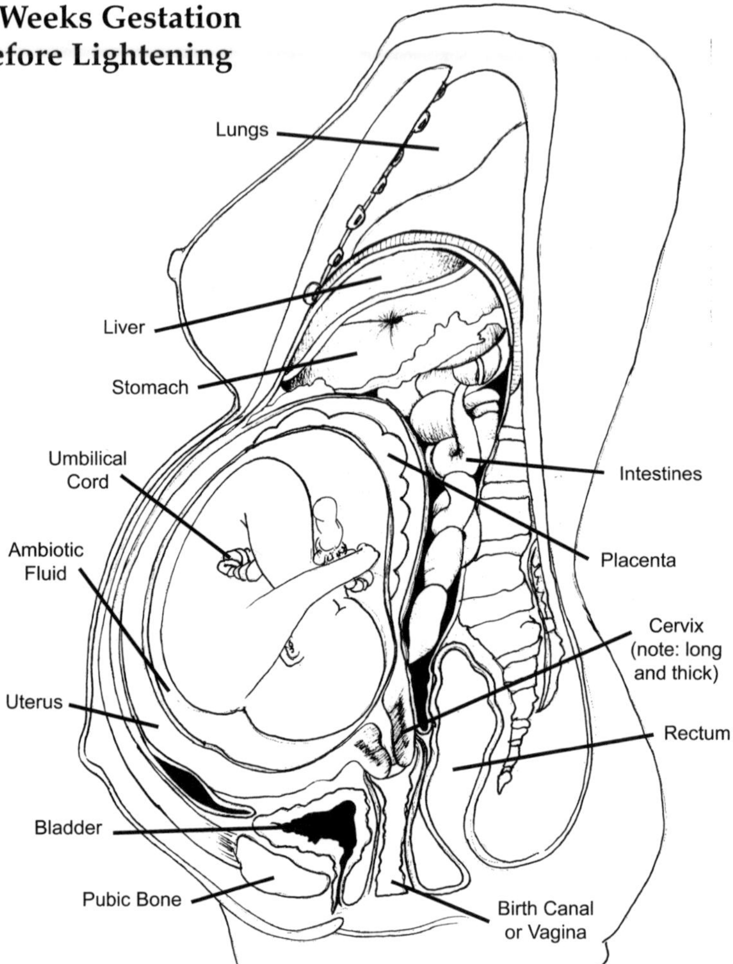

Drawn by Molly Harrison

The diagram above shows the uterus at 36 weeks gestation before lightening, which is when the baby drops down into the pelvis. Locate all the labeled body parts. Now, notice how high the baby is positioned and how all your organs (stomach, liver, lungs) are pushed together. This compact feeling forces you to eat small, frequent meals. You may also feel like you have trouble taking a deep breath. When sleeping, you will be using lots of pillows to position yourself in order to breathe and relax. Good news: notice how much room your bladder has. In this first

36 Weeks Gestation After Lightening

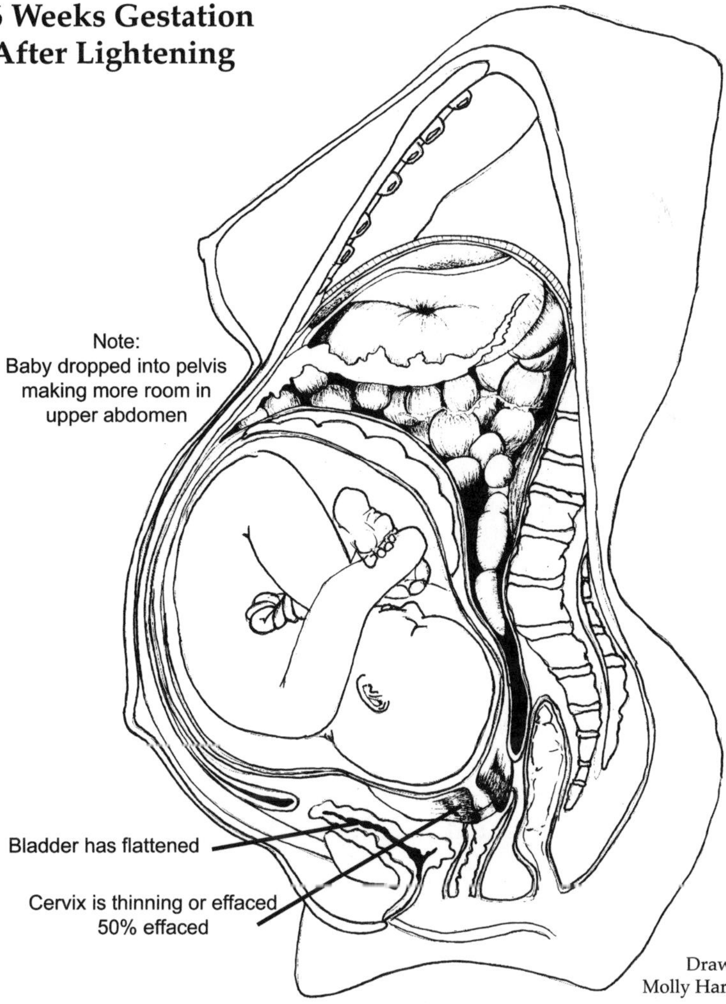

Drawn by
Molly Harrison

diagram, the opening of the uterus, called your cervix, is thick and approximately 1½ inches long. Review at 36 weeks before lightening: uterus, placenta, cord, amniotic fluid, fundus, cervix.

The diagram above shows the uterus at 36 weeks gestation after lightening. Notice that the cervix is thinning or effacing; it's about 50 percent effaced. Compare previous diagram and note how low the baby is located in the pelvis, leaving more room for stomach and lungs for breathing—but look at the bladder. You will experience frequent bathroom visits, as well as pelvic fullness.

Warning Signs During Late Pregnancy

Call your healthcare provider if you are experiencing any of the following:

- Contractions before thirty-seven weeks
- Rupture of membranes – leaking or a gushing of fluid from the vagina
- Fever greater than 101
- Blurred vision, spots before your eyes
- Swelling of face
- Headaches
- Vaginal bleeding
- Vomiting
- Burning or pain with urination

Other non-emergency issues that may cause discomfort, such as constipation, can be addressed and answered during regular office hours. Your doctor, midwife or nurse practitioner may also give you a list of medications that are approved to take if needed.

Labor and Birth

The more you learn about how your body works during labor, the better you can utilize comfort measures and positions to help ease the pain, enhance your labor pattern, and build your confidence. Many women stress about their ability to stay in control during labor or they have a fear of losing control. This fear can be calmed by changing your mindset from worrying about "losing control" to surrendering to the labor and trusting your own body as you allow it to do its work.

One of the responsibilities of your support person is to create an atmosphere that is conducive to laboring. This may be achieved by walking with you, giving back rubs, providing light foods and fluids, watching your favorite movie together, helping with packing your luggage or suggesting a warm shower or bath.

Focus on relaxing and concentrate on listening to your body. As your labor progresses, your support person(s) should try to create a calming environment by dimming the lights, playing your favorite music, or just sitting quietly by your side.

The Four Stages of Labor

Stage 1

The first stage of labor is divided into three phases: early, active and transitional. Labor begins when contractions occur at regular intervals or a spontaneous rupture of the membrane of the amniotic sac (commonly referred to as *the breaking of the waters*) and continues as the contractions last longer, become more frequent, and are strong enough to completely dilate and efface your cervix. Dilation is the opening of the cervix from closed to 10 centimeters. Effacement is the thinning and flattening out of the cervix. At 100 percent effacement, the cervix is paper-thin and at 10 centimeters dilation, you are ready to begin the pushing phase.

Stage 2

The second stage of labor begins with complete dilation and effacement of the cervix, and lasts until the birth of the baby.

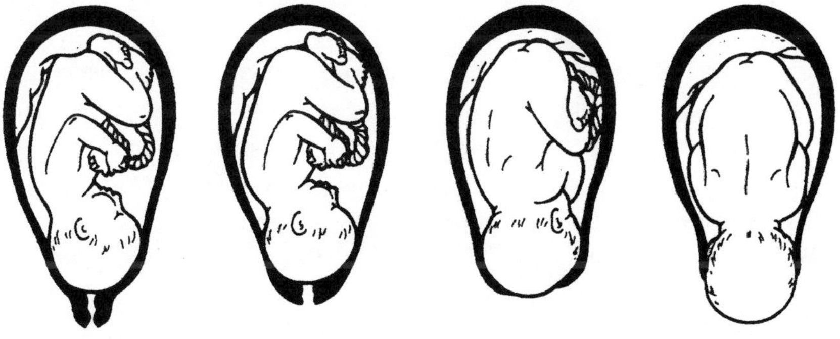

none	50%	90%	100%
none	2–3 cm	5 cm	9 cm

Stage 3

The third stage begins with birth of baby, and lasts until the placenta is delivered.

Stage 4

The fourth stage begins once the placenta is delivered and lasts until the end of the first hour of recovery.

I will start with the first stage of labor and review in greater detail the emotional and physical changes you may experience, as well as which comfort measures may be helpful during each stage.

The first stage of labor is divided into three phases:

- Phase one— latent or early labor (Some refer to this as home labor)
- Phase two— active labor
- Phase three— transitional labor

Phase One—Latent or Early Labor

In the last few weeks of your pregnancy, your cervix will become soft, also known as ripening. This means that labor could be soon approaching or weeks away. Your cervix will begin to shorten or efface as well as open or dilate. Many healthcare providers will do pelvic examinations starting at 36 weeks gestation. They will also take a vaginal culture for Group B Strep infection (see glossary). If this culture is positive, you will be given antibiotics while you are in labor to protect your baby from contracting this bacteria.

You may feel your uterus tightening throughout your pregnancy, especially notable the last few weeks. This tightening is called Braxton Hicks contractions, sometimes referred to as "false labor" or "practice labor." These contractions don't cause any changes in the cervix and will not have the three characteristics of contractions for true labor. Real, true labor contractions become stronger, last longer and come closer together.

Note: Even a little dehydration can cause Braxton Hicks contractions. If you have been busy all day or working outside in the yard, and have not had enough water to drink, these contractions can easily occur. Drink a large glass of water and lie on your left side. These Braxton Hicks contractions will subside.

True contractions will be mild in intensity, lasting only 30 to 45 seconds in duration, and will be anywhere from 5 to 20 minutes apart. Many women will experience these mild, menstrual-like cramps and continue to go about their day until the intensity of the contractions increases.

Don't start timing too soon. Wait until you can't walk or talk through your contractions to begin timing them. In the meantime, if it's nighttime, try to get sleep. If you can't sleep, let your partner sleep unless you need the extra support. If you aren't comfortable lying down, get up and move around the house. Watch your favorite movie, walk, lean over the kitchen counter, sit on the birth ball, and get on your hands and knees. If your back hurts, take a warm shower or bath. Get something light to eat, drink a cup of warm tea, or call your doula to ask for other suggestions. Most importantly, rest if you can.

Only one out of ten women have their membranes rupture (their water breaks) before contractions begin or during the early phase of labor, after contractions have been established. Ask your healthcare provider what she wishes for you to do if your membranes do rupture. Some healthcare providers want you at the hospital sooner rather than later while others will allow you to stay at home until labor is well established.

When your contractions become more regular—meaning, they are lasting longer, stronger and coming closer together—you will start timing them.

How to Time and Evaluate a Contraction

Duration: This tells you how long the contraction lasts. Measuring in seconds, you will note when the contraction (or tightening of the uterus) begins and when it is over (or the uterus is relaxed).

Once your contractions become strong enough for timing, you will most likely find them to be about 30 to 45 seconds, increasing in duration to 60 to 90 seconds.

Interval: This tells you how far apart the contractions are. This time begins ***at the start of one contraction to the beginning of the next contraction, <u>not</u> from the end of one to the beginning of the next.***

In early labor, the contractions will be anywhere from 5 to 20 minutes apart. Few women start with contractions less than 5 minutes apart and extremely intense.

5-20 minutes intervals

Intensity: When you find that you can't walk or talk through each contraction, the level of intensity has increased. Remember that your body knows what to do. Relax with each contraction and let your body do its work. At this time, you may need to use your relaxed breathing pattern. Between contractions, you will feel completely fine. Use this time to pack your bags, make important phone calls, bake the baby a birthday cake, or cookies for a snack later and for sharing with your support team and/or nursing staff, play your favorite music, and write down your feelings of excitement and anticipation of your new arrival. You may wish for your partner, doula or other support person to be present as the contractions become stronger, longer and closer together.

As the contractions become stronger, many women begin to worry that birth is close. Fathers and partners may begin to worry that they will be delivering the baby in the living room, or worse, in the car! Relax. You will have plenty of time. Usually if you are having a precipitous delivery (a labor and birth less than 3 hours), your contractions will begin close together (2 minutes apart) and will be very intense. The average first labor is 15 to 20 hours. So, again, relax. Trust your body, welcome each contraction, and enjoy the quiet moments between each one.

When to Call Your Doctor or Midwife

Your doctor or midwife will usually give you specific instructions as you get closer to your due date. Most will tell you to call when your contractions are 4 to 5 minutes apart, lasting 60 seconds, and you can no longer walk or talk through them. You will need to check in with your doctor or midwife if your water breaks, especially if you tested positive for Group B Strep. Most women just need to remember **5-1-1** or **4-1-1**. This means that your contractions are **4 to 5 minutes** apart, lasting **one** minute for at least **one** hour. If you live close to the hospital or birthing center, they may instruct you to wait until the contractions are 3 to 4 minutes apart.

Ask yourself whether you would rather labor at home with familiar things in a quiet environment or if you'd prefer to get to the hospital too soon, just to find yourself sitting around, being denied food, hooked up to a fetal monitoring system. Again, **trust your body; trust yourself. You can do it.** Have your support partner/team nearby during this time. Don't panic. Think positive about the birth journey you are experiencing. The sooner the contractions become stronger, last longer and occur closer together, the sooner your beautiful baby will arrive.

What to Bring to the Hospital

You may have many of these items gathered together in a corner of your room, just waiting for the first sign of labor before packing. During early labor, between contractions is a good time to finish packing your needed items. Here is a list of suggested items you may wish to bring to the hospital or birthing center.

- Birth Plan
- Insurance Card
- Picture ID (required by most hospitals)
- Cell phone and charger
- Telephone calling card if your family and friends are long distance and you don't have or will not be using a cell phone

- Laptop computer—many hospitals have wireless internet
- Focal Point— A focal point is an object or particular item in the room—it might be something such as a small picture, stuffed animal, religious icon, object of power, anything that speaks to you personally that you want to use to focus attention to or concentrate on during your contractions. Some women find having a focal point helps them get through each contraction, and others do not.
- Camera with extra batteries/charger or extra film if needed
- Music—CD player or iPod loaded with your favorite music
- Snacks for partner/possible fruit pops for you or vitamin water
- Birth ball if hospital doesn't have three or four
- Lip balm
- Your own clothes for laboring if you do not want to wear a hospital gown
- Robe and slippers
- Warm socks
- Tennis balls or massagers
- Toothbrush/toothpaste and mouthwash, as well as partner's oral hygiene gear
- Favorite lotion
- Aromatherapy—mom's favorite—but NO **candles** or incense. Karla's favorite recipe:
  Sprinkle 3 drops of lavender and 1 drop of peppermint into a bowl of cold water, stir, then use a washcloth dipped in this mix as a forehead compress.
- Massage oil with jasmine, neroli, rose and lavender
- Coins for vending machines
- List of important phone numbers. If you have a large number of people to call, make a phone tree beforehand, having each person on the tree call the next, so that this task doesn't take you away from bonding with your new baby.
- Pad of paper or journal and a pen for recording the day's events

Hospital Bag

- Night gowns (2-3)
- Nursing bras (2-3)
- Toiletries for both mom/partner
- Makeup/hairdryer
- Going home clothes for mom and baby
- Change of clothes for partner
- Receiving blanket/warm clothes for baby if winter
- Car seat for baby, already installed in car

Once your labor is well established and you are ready to leave for the hospital or birthing center, be sure to call your doctor or midwife. They may need to call the hospital or birthing center to let the nursing staff know to expect you. If the place where you are planning to give birth has only one or two tubs, and you wish to use it as a comfort measure, let your midwife know you will want to use the tub when you call. This way, the nurse can assign you to the labor room with the tub if it's available.

During your pregnancy, you should take a tour of the hospital or birthing center where you plan to give birth so you will be familiar with the surroundings, such as where to park and where to enter the building at what times. The entrance place can change depending on the time of day. Entering the hospital or birthing center with all your items will decrease any chance of your support person needing to leave you alone.

Once in the labor and delivery suite, many routine procedures occur. Most of these procedures are your doctor's orders. This is why it is important to have your birth plan reviewed by your doctor and have her give your plan her "blessing" in advance. The first things that typically happen are that a nurse will ask you to change your clothes, empty your bladder, and get into bed for 20 to 30 minutes of fetal monitoring. If this feels and sounds comfortable and okay, then do it.

If this stresses you a bit, then get your birth plan out of the bag and review the things that are important to you. If your birth plan states that you wish to wear your own clothes, insist.

Wearing your own clothes may keep you calm and not feeling like a patient. This is one instance where your support person is important. Between contractions, your support person is getting out the birth plan, finding your labor clothes, setting up your music, and arranging the room to create a soothing, calm environment as close as possible to the kind you may have had at home.

Many women like to sit in a rocking chair during fetal monitoring. Fetal monitoring is the recording of your contractions simultaneously with your baby's heart rate. Two belts will be placed around your belly to hold the circular monitoring devices in place. The top device will record the contractions while the lower device monitors and records the baby's heart rate.

If you are experiencing back labor, you will be more comfortable standing with your upper body across the bed or leaning over the birth ball while on your hands and knees. Again, most nurses don't mind where you sit or stand, or how you labor, just as long as they are able to get a good period of fetal monitoring to show how the baby is reacting to the contractions. If all is well,

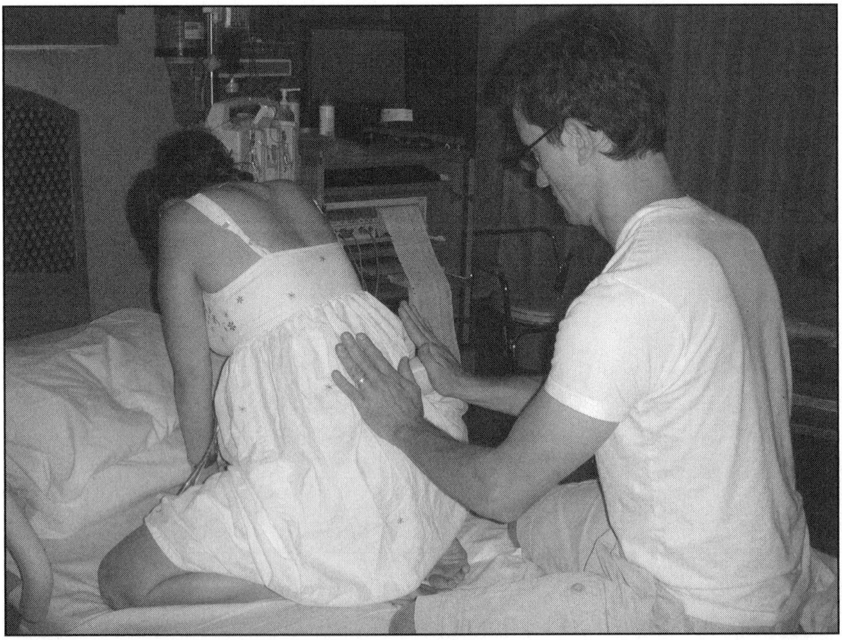

Brian helps Dee's back pain by providing counter-pressure on her back.

most hospitals will allow you to have intermittent electronic fetal monitoring, which is 20 minutes of monitoring out of every hour. This is a doctor's order, so be sure to discuss the issue of monitoring with your doctor. Many midwives will use a hand-held fetal monitoring device called a Doppler during and after a few contractions to check on the baby's well-being.

During your admission to the labor suite and while being monitored, the nurse will ask you questions concerning your medical history regarding this pregnancy, past family medical history, and whether or not you have any special needs or requests. The nurse will have you sign several permission forms giving your healthcare provider and the hospital staff permission to treat you and the baby. These forms will also give permission for the use of anesthesia if needed or requested, and gives permission to circumcise your son if you choose to have that procedure done. All of this is done between contractions, so your partner needs to be by your side, helping with comfort measures that work during this time. Remember, the sooner the admission

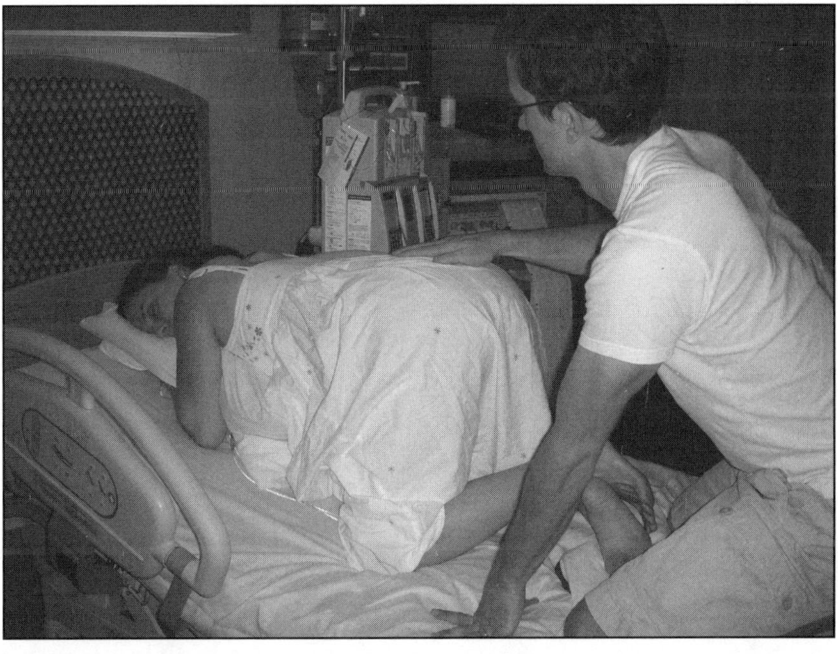

This hands and knees position aids with rotating the posterior baby.

process is completed, the sooner you can get disconnected from the fetal monitoring belts and move freely around the room.

After the first period of fetal monitoring, your doctor, midwife or nurse may wish to check your cervix for any progress. They will also be checking the station of your baby which is the position of the presenting part (baby's head) in relationship to your ischial spines which are the bones marking the middle of the true pelvis. This is an exciting time, especially if the cervix has made big changes. It can also be a bit discouraging if little progress is noted.

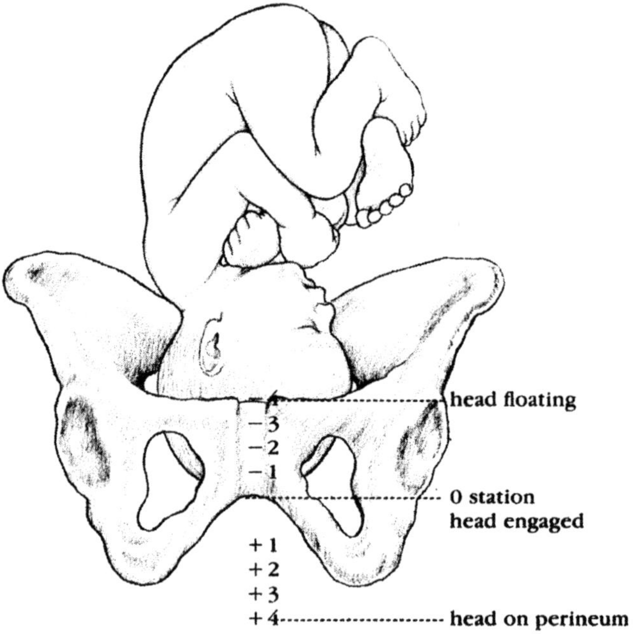

Stations of descent

As a doula, I think this can be a very tough time for many women. But remember, it's all part of your birth journey. Why is this moment tough? Well, let's say you are 40 weeks gestation. At your last doctor or midwife visit, your cervix was 50 percent effaced and 1 centimeter dilated. You have labored at home for 10 hours. Your contractions are 4 minutes apart, lasting 60 seconds, very intense. After checking your cervix, the report is that you are 1 to 2 centimeters and 80 to 90 percent effaced. You were just sure you were at least 6 centimeters. Your partner was sure you were farther along, too, as he looks at you and exclaims, "Is that all?!" Now, now, don't kill him, you'll need him later. You might feel as though you've made hardly any progress at all. Are you really in good labor? Yes, yes, yes!

It takes the body time to get into a pattern of good, strong contractions that cause dilating and effacing of the cervix. It can take up to 10 hours just to thin out the cervix. At 80 to 90 percent effaced, a cervix will start dilating faster. Instead of feeling disheartened, focus on encouraging your body to continue this work. Walk, slow dance, relax, listen to music, get a hug and get refocused on the journey.

If you are in early labor, many midwives will allow you to go home if your membranes aren't ruptured. Most doctors will keep you since you are already there. If you go into labor during the day, call your doctor or midwife's office first—you may be able to go by and be checked. This may allow you to delay the hospital admission. The longer you are in the hospital, the greater the chances that you will have to receive interventions.

During Early Labor

- **Fluids:** Drink to quench thirst, and eat if you are hungry. You will feel better if you stay hydrated, but you don't need to over hydrate. Eat easily digested foods like bagel and cream cheese, soups, toast and jam or peanut butter, eggs, pancakes, bananas, applesauce, yogurt, etc. Especially while you are at home, eat foods that sound good to you and have lots of protein and carbohydrates which give you strength for later when you may not feel like eating anything or will not have access to food in the hospital.

- **Comfort measures:** During this early labor, you will listen to your body, rest if you can, walk, go shopping, watch a favorite movie or listen to music, rock, lean over the birth ball, get on your hands and knees to do lower back stretches if your back aches, or use the shower.

Comfort Measures...whatever works

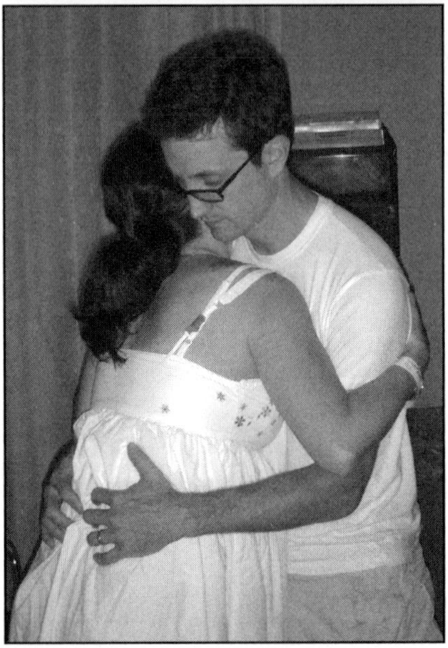

Slow dancing is a wonderful way to pass time in labor.

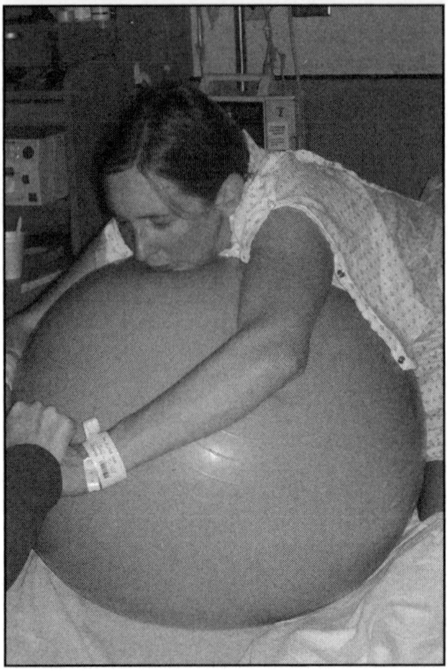

Birth balls are great for sitting or leaning over, giving the mother's arms and legs a rest.

- **Vaginal checks:** This will occur when entering the hospital or birthing center for a baseline of cervical changes.

- **Partner's role:** Be supportive by listening to her requests. Go walking or shopping with her. Encourage her to rest if possible, eat and drink. That includes you, also.

- **Doula's role:** Call your doula and let her know you are in early labor. She should be able to give you suggestions on comfort measures. Many doulas come to your home and help you when the contractions become intense or when you need support.

Phase Two—Active Labor

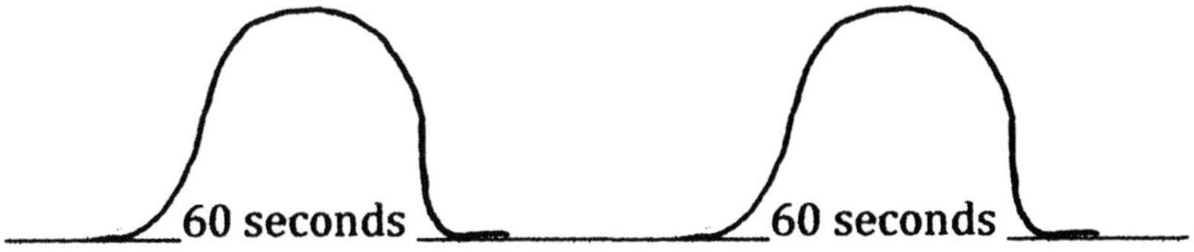

2-4 minute intervals

During the active phase of labor, you will have very intense contractions, 2 to 4 minutes apart, and lasting 60 seconds or longer, for an average of 3 to 5 hours while your cervix dilates 4 to 7 centimeters.

You will need support and help with staying focused. You will also need your support person to help keep the room a calm place and conducive for laboring. This may be a time when all visitors need to leave. Since the contractions will increase with intensity, it may be necessary to use some different comfort measures. If you are managing well, great, continue with what you are doing. If you are having trouble finding a comfortable place or a relaxing position, try the shower or tub. It can bring great relief and can increase relaxation. According to Barbara Harper's book *Gentle Births,* studies have shown that submerging your belly in water during labor can give you the same pain relief as a shot of narcotics without the undesirable side-effects. Most doctors agree that a laboring woman can spend 40 to 90 minutes in a warm tub, then get out for 20 minutes of monitoring, and then return to the tub, if she so desires. Midwives use a handheld Doppler while you remain in the tub.

Some women feel very trapped during this phase. They may be tired if labor has been going on for hours. They get discouraged and think they can't go on much longer. Many women will ask for medication. If her plan is low intervention, then work with her through these few moments. Her body will increase its own endorphins (pain relief) and the contractions will seem more manageable.

Encouragement from everyone in the labor room is vital. Acknowledge her pain and hard work. Tell her that she is strong and to trust her body. Surrender to the labor and allow her body to do its work. Stay relaxed and change breathing patterns if needed.

During Active Labor

- **Fluids:** Most hospitals and birthing centers will allow you to have clear liquids like water, tea, Gatorade, vitamin water, ginger ale, ice pops, ice chips, or Jell-O to stay hydrated. You can take small sips between contractions to replenish fluids. Most hospitals like for you to have an IV (intravenous), or at least a saline lock, a small, plastic catheter in your vein, which is capped off and taped. This way, IV fluids can quickly be administered if an emergency arises.

- **Comfort measures:** Listen to your body. What position is comfortable for you? Upright positions, relaxation, breathing

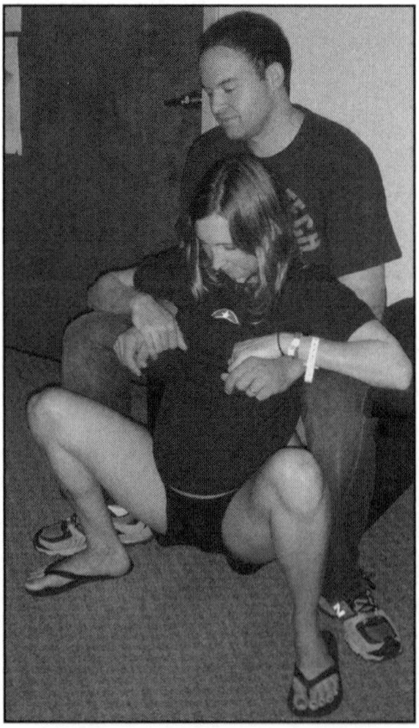
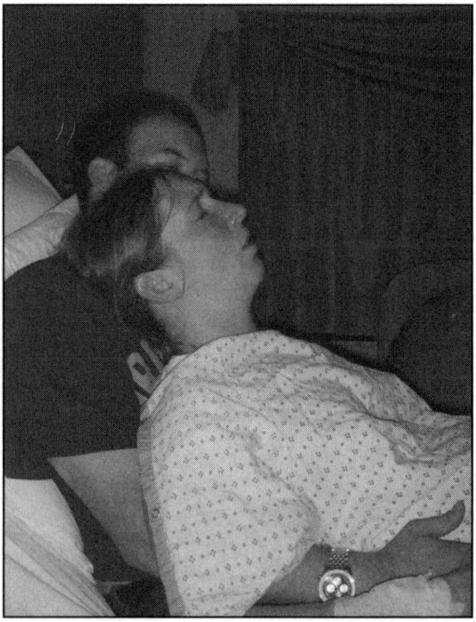

Allison found the squatting position during labor very helpful. Jeremy provided strength and support.

techniques, slow dancing, walking, rocking chair, sitting on the toilet or birth ball, squatting, shower/tub, on your hands and knees or leaning over the back of the bed.

- **Vaginal checks:** Either your doctor, midwife or nurse will do the initial vaginal exam. After that, you will only be checked if you request medication, if your labor pattern doesn't progress in a timely fashion, if you feel the urge to push, or if your membrane ruptures. After your water breaks, a vaginal check is performed to assure that the baby's head is tight against the cervix and the umbilical cord hasn't slipped out in front of the baby and gets pinched off by the baby's head (known as a prolapsed cord).

- **Partner's role:** After getting mom settled in the labor and delivery suite, or the birthing center, the partner should be sure to give the birth plan to the nurse, then help mom to relax and get focused on the contractions. Create a calm atmosphere in the room by dimming the lights and adding her favorite music. Be mom's advocate. Sit by her side. Give her a hug

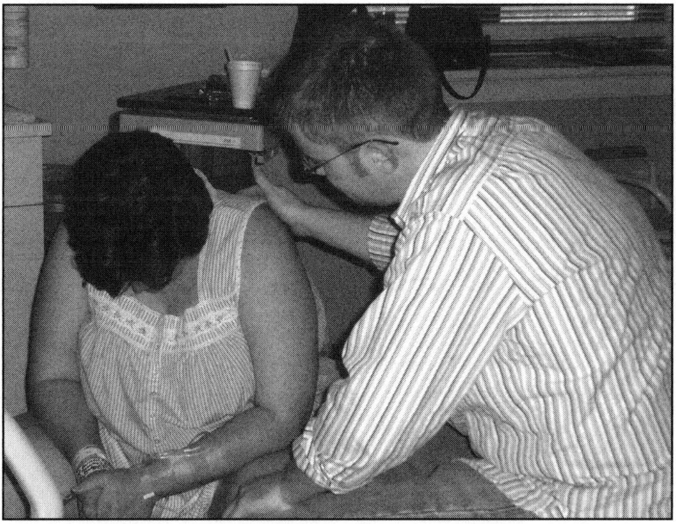

Jennifer loved when Ger sat next to her and stayed close during contractions.

and kiss. Tell her how excited you are and how strong she is. During this time, don't forget to take care of yourself. Be sure to eat and drink as needed.

- **Doula's role:** She will help the mother get into the most comfortable positions, get ice chips, fill the tub with water, get the partner any needed fluids, help mother with breathing patterns in order to get her relaxed and focused, as well as provide a calm presence.

Phase Three—Transitional Labor

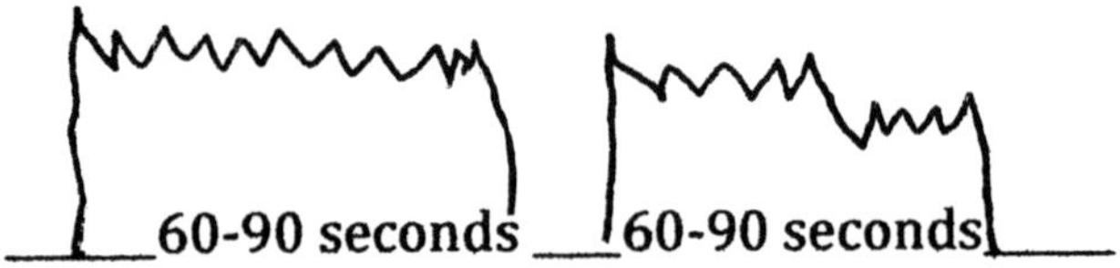

30 seconds to 1½ minutes

During this phase of labor, your contractions will occur every 1 to 2 minutes and will continue to feel intense. This phase usually lasts between 30 to 90 minutes. Since there is little rest time between contractions, you may begin to feel very overwhelmed. A calm, quiet atmosphere and good, continuous support are essential.

Due to the hard work the body is doing, hiccups, burping, waves of nausea, uncontrollable shaking, and occasional vomiting are common for some women. As the baby moves down deeper into the pelvis, you may feel "butt" pressure. This can be very intense, especially at the peak of the contraction. It is best to get your doctor, midwife or nurse to check your cervix when you have this bearing down pressure during and after a contraction. You may be fully dilated and ready to start pushing. You don't want to push if your cervix isn't fully dilated. Pushing too soon can cause cervical swelling.

During Transitional Labor

- **Comfort measures:** Since contractions are intense, you may find comfort in the warm tub or shower, moving around in upright positions, sitting on a birth ball or just lying on your side in the bed. You will want the room to be quiet, possibly with soft music, and you will want any talking or movement by others in the room to be kept to a minimum.

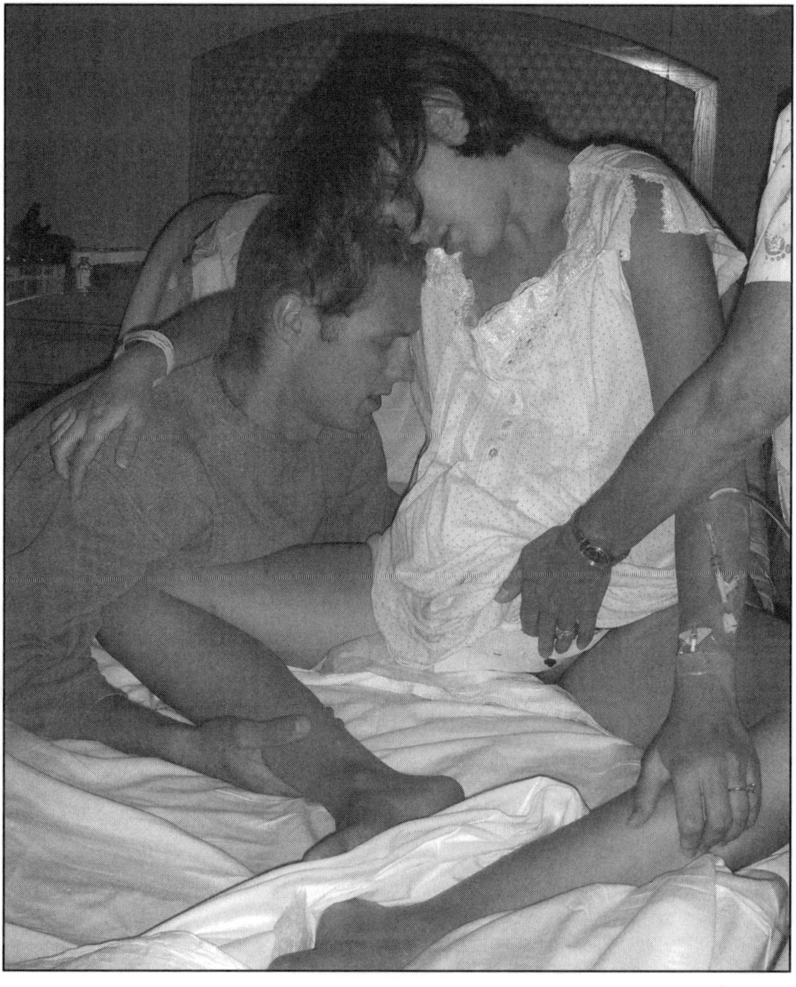

Stephanie receives strength and support from Michael during the challenges of transitional labor.

- **Vaginal checks:** Vaginal exams will be kept to a minimum. If you have the urge to push, the doctor, midwife, or nurse will check to see if you are dilated to 10 centimeters and whether you are ready to push.

- **Partner's role:** Stay by mom's side. Helping with back pressure, breathing pattern, focus point, offering ice chips, cool cloths, anything to help support her and meet her needs. If you need a rest, take a quick break in the room. Don't leave mom by herself at this time.

- **Doula's role:** To help with comfort measures, make suggestions for position changes if needed, offer ice chips, help with breathing and focus, especially if partner needs a break. Be by the mother's side. The doula should never leave the room during this time.

The Second Stage of Labor

begins with complete dilation and effacement of cervix until the birth of the baby.

Let the Pushing Begin!

When this stage begins, many women will notice that the contractions will slow a bit, occurring every 2 to 5 minutes. This gives you a break. Rest between contractions to gain strength for the pushing. Pushing the baby down the birth canal may take less than 30 minutes, especially for second time mothers, or it may take as long as 4 hours. The length of time also depends on how high the baby is in the pelvis (also known as station of baby) when pushing begins, and on whether or not you have an epidural anesthesia.

During the Second Stage of Labor

- **Positions for pushing:** If you are unmedicated, you can push standing, squatting, sitting on the toilet, semi-sitting, side-lying, or on your hands and knees. If you have an epidural, you will most likely push in the semi-sitting or side-lying position.

- **Comfort measures:** Your support person(s) will help you get into a good position for optimal pushing. They will continue to offer ice chips and cool cloths to place across your forehead or on the back of your neck.

- **Vaginal checks:** The only reason vaginal checks are done during this time is to check the station of your baby's progress after pushing for an hour or so.

- **Partner's role:** To offer ice chips between contractions, a cool cloth, to support mom's legs, especially if she has an epidural, and to provide encouraging words.

- **Doula's role:** About the same as the partner, ice chips, cool cloth, supporting mom's legs during pushing. And between contractions, helping the mother to relax and rest.

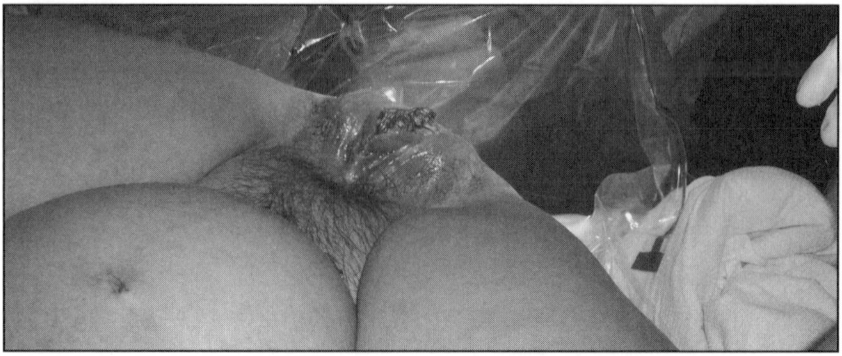

After a few minutes of pushing, Lula's head is crowning.

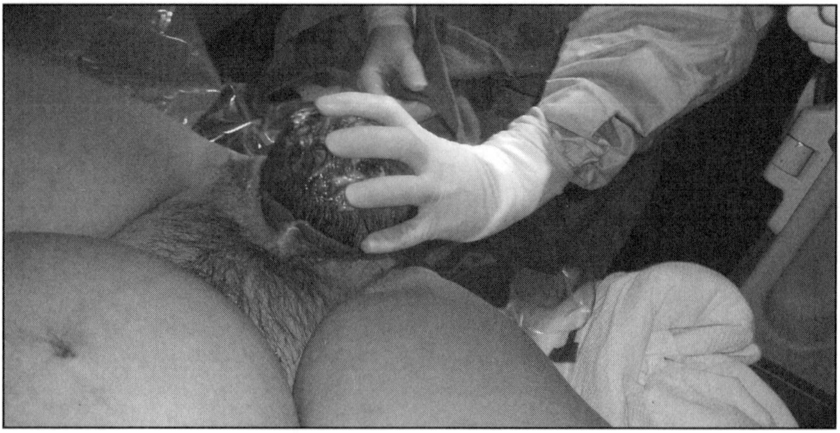

Her head is slowly guided out…

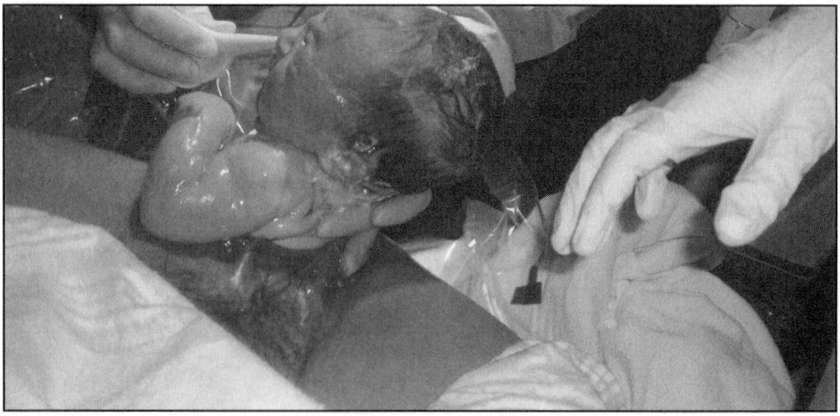

…then her shoulder.

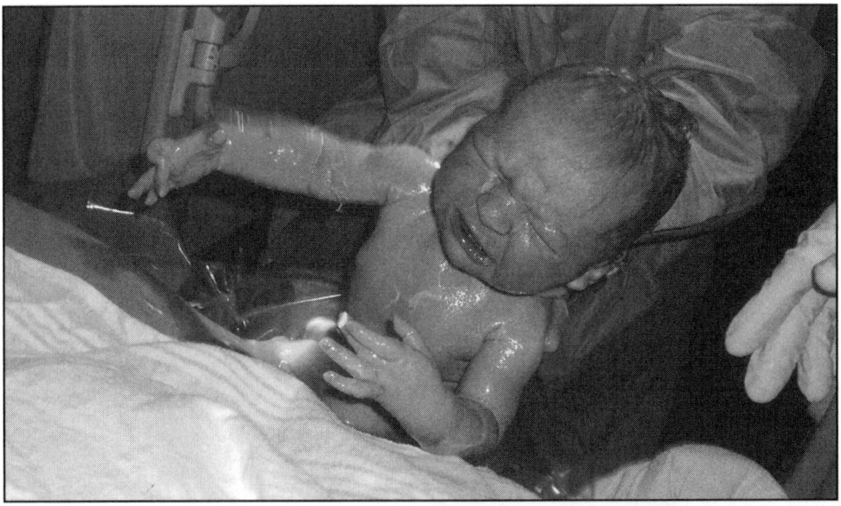

She has arrived!

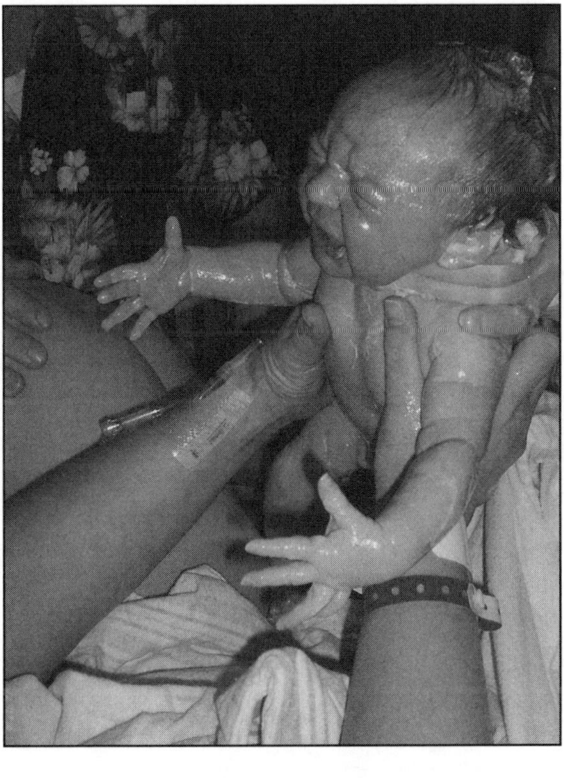

As Lula's body emerges, Karla reaches for her beautiful baby girl.

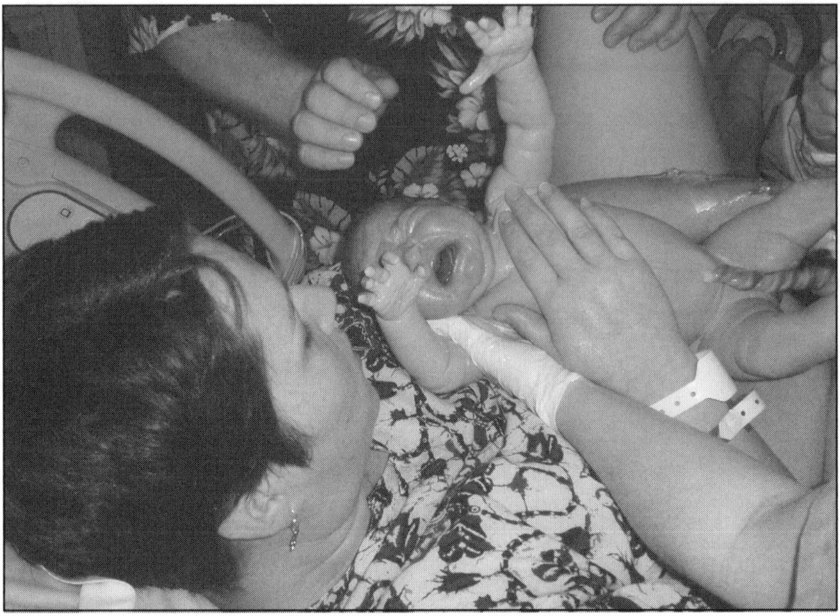

Lula is placed on Karla's chest.

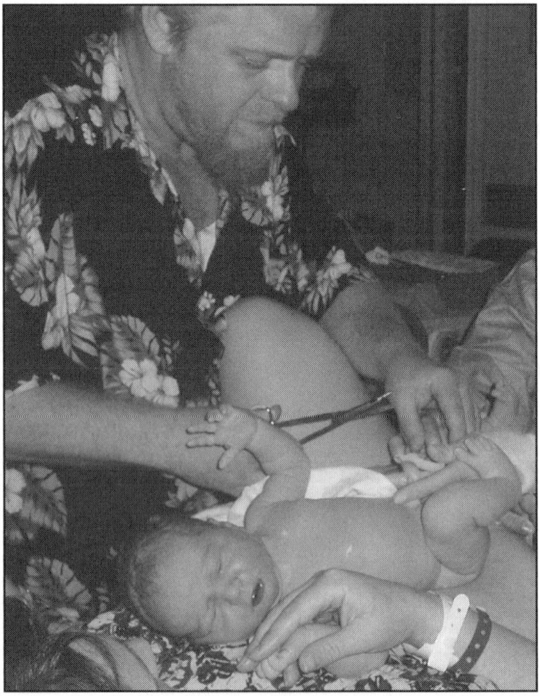

Jamie cuts her umbilical cord.

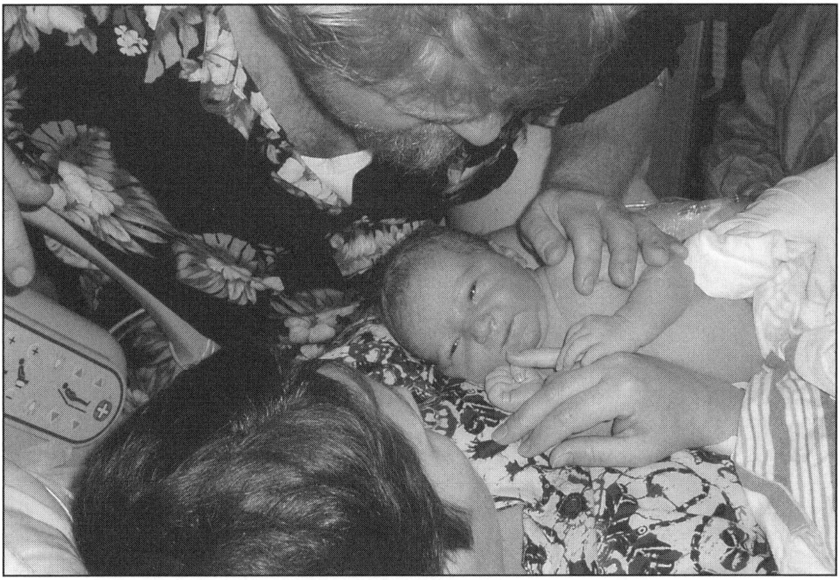

Bonding time begins.

The Third Stage of Labor
begins with birth of baby and lasts until
the placenta is delivered.

The placenta will detach from the wall of the uterus to be expelled through the birth canal. This process takes from 10 to 30 minutes. There is a lull in the intensity of contractions after the birth of the baby. This stage is very short and the least painful of all the stages. During this time, your healthcare provider will repair any lacerations or tears if needed.

During the Third Stage of Labor

- **Comfort measures:** Continuing to have your legs supported if needed, getting fresh clothes, have pillows placed under your arms for support while holding your beautiful, new baby.

- **Partner's role:** To bond with baby while he or she rests on mother's chest, praise mom and share your excitement.

- **Doula's role:** To be present to help with any requests, remind mother of breathing with contractions and explain any procedures if she needs you to do so. Take pictures of the new family!

The Fourth Stage of Labor

begins after the placenta is removed and continues throughout the first hour of recovery.

During this first hour, your blood pressure will be taken frequently, the fundus (top of uterus) will be massaged to assure it stays firm and, to decrease any chance of hemorrhage, ice will be placed on your perineal area, and food and drink will be provided.

During the Fourth Stage of Labor

- **Comfort measures:** Have help to get into a comfortable position for nursing your baby for the first time, getting something to eat and drink, using the bathroom or taking a shower.

- **Partner's role:** To continue holding and bonding with baby, taking pictures, getting a snack.

- **Doula's role:** To praise mom for a job well done. To be present to aid in any request, bring food or drink. Help with breastfeeding, help mom with showering or using the bathroom.

Now that we have discussed the four stages of labor and the role of the partner and doula, it is important to understand the common interventions that are used during labor and birth.

Interventions

Electronic Fetal Monitoring

As mentioned earlier, this type of monitoring tells your healthcare provider how well your baby is tolerating your contractions by recording the baby's heart rate and simultaneously recording your contractions. This is usually done upon arrival at the hospital while the nurse is admitting you. Soft, elastic belts are used to keep an external monitor around your belly. If, for whatever reason, a good external fetal monitor tracing isn't obtained, then an internal scalp electrode will be attached to the fetus's head. Your cervix needs to be 2 to 3 centimeters dilated and your amniotic membranes must be ruptured before internal monitoring can be done. For external monitoring, most healthcare providers will allow you to be intermittently monitored for 20 minutes or less out of every hour if the recording looks good. You will need continuous monitoring if you are receiving Pitocin or epidural anesthesia. I explain both of these in greater detail below.

Intravenous Fluids

A small plastic tube, called an "IV," is placed in a vein in your arm that allows for fluids to be administered in case of an emergency, if you request the use of epidural anesthesia, or if you are unable to maintain hydration due to nausea and vomiting. Many healthcare providers will allow you to have a "saline lock," sometimes called a "hep-lock." This means that the nurse will place a small amount of normal saline (heparin was previously used, but is used no longer) in the tubing close to your IV insertion site, and then will disconnect the tubing from the bag of fluid. This allows you to walk freely without having to push the IV pole. You can also easily get into and out of the shower or tub.

Pitocin

This is a synthetic form of oxytocin, used to stimulate contractions or to augment contractions. This drug is administered by IV and you must remain continuously on the fetal monitor since some babies react negatively to high doses of this drug. If you are planning to be induced, Pitocin is one of the medications needed. Side effects of Pitocin are fetal distress caused by intensely strong uterine contractions that last too long or contractions not subsiding completely to allow good exchange of oxygen during the time between contractions. There is a much higher incidence of uterine rupture especially if given at a high rate or used with VBAC (vaginal birth after cesarean) births.

Amniotomy

During this procedure your healthcare provider will rupture your amniotic sac (or bag of water) using an instrument with a tiny, sharp tip that looks like a plastic knitting needle. It feels like having a vaginal exam. After your membranes are ruptured, amniotic fluid will continuously leak, so you will need to wear a sanitary pad and panties if you are up and walking around. This procedure may be done if you are being induced and your cervix is 2 or more centimeters dilated, or if you have a fever during labor and examination of the fluid is needed. Some doctors will rupture your membranes in order to stimulate contractions. According to Michael Benson's book *Obstetrical Pearls: A Practical Guide for the Efficient Resident,* studies have shown that rupturing the membranes does not shorten labor time. Doing so will increase the intensity of the contractions since the cushion of water on the cervix is removed. Once your membranes are ruptured (either naturally or by your healthcare provider), you may be restricted from using the tub due to concerns that immersion in water may result in an increased risk of infection. Showering is usually considered safe with ruptured membranes. After membranes have ruptured, many healthcare providers put your labor "on the clock," wanting either a vaginal or caesarean-section birth (also known as C-section or C-birth) within 12 to 24 hours. Since the amniotic membrane protects your baby from the outside world, many healthcare providers want you to deliver as soon as possible. If infection is a concern, antibiotics can be started.

Medically Assisted Births

Use of Forceps

Forceps are a metal instrument resembling tongs that are placed on each side of the baby's head once the baby is in the birth canal, and are used to assist in removing the baby from the birth canal. The mother must push as the doctor guides the baby out. This instrument would be used when the baby is experiencing fetal distress while in the birth canal and needs immediate delivery. They may also be used if the mother has lost all sensation of pushing, due to numbing from epidural anesthesia, and needs assistance. Redness or bruising on the baby's cheek area may be present for several days after birth, due to pressure of the forceps.

Vacuum Extractor

This small rubber suction cup is placed on the top of your baby's head when the baby is in the birth canal in order to assist the mother with delivery. The mother still must push as the healthcare provider guides the baby out. This instrument can leave bruising and small cuts on top of the baby's head.

Episiotomy

This is a small incision made on the perineum either straight downward from the vaginal opening toward the rectum or off to one side. It is performed to enlarge the birth canal. According to the Cochrone Review, this procedure is no longer routine since scientific studies in the 1990s have found no benefits and some real risks to routine episiotomy.

Medications During Labor

Analgesics

Analgesics are used for pain relief. Two common analgesics used in labor are Stadol and Nubain. Both are narcotics. These medicines work by changing your perception of pain and "takes the edge off." You will still feel some pain or discomfort with contractions. Many women experience disorientation, dizziness, nausea, lowered blood pressure, itching and occasionally, vomiting. Analgesics will not be given too close to birth since the baby will also receive the effects of the medications, which can affect their ability to breathe upon delivery. Narcan can be given to counteract this negative side effect if necessary. Many breastfed babies have feeding issues the first 24 hours after birth, usually due to uncoordinated suck, if their mothers have received either of these narcotics during labor.

Epidural Anesthesia

This form of anesthesia is commonly used in this country for pain relief for labor as well as anesthesia for Caesarean births (C-birth). A mixture of narcotics and anesthetic (numbing) medications are administered through a small catheter placed by an anesthesiologist into the dura (the outside covering of the spinal column) on the lower part of your back. The catheter is securely taped onto your back and then connected to a continuous drip of the mix of medications. There are advantages and disadvantages for using epidural during labor.

Advantages:

- Provides the mother with pain relief from the contractions.
- Allows the mother to rest if labor is prolonged.
- Allows the mother to be awake during a C-birth so that she can hear her baby's first cry and can see and touch her baby during the surgery.

- Provides pain relief if assisted delivery instruments are used, or for repair of an episiotomy, if one is performed.

Disadvantages:

- Restricts the laboring mother to bed with limited mobility.
- During administration, a temporary drop in maternal blood pressure may occur. Epinephrine can be given to correct this problem.
- If given too early in labor, an epidural may slow or even stop contractions, which will require the use of additional administration of medications like Pitocin.
- Electronic fetal monitoring and pulse oximeter (a non-invasive rubber attachment on the mother's finger to monitor her breathing and oxygen level) must be used continuously.
- Epidural usually increases the use of other interventions during the second stage of labor (pushing phase), such as the use of forceps or a vacuum extractor.
- Since the bladder will also be numbed by the epidural medicine, it's difficult to empty your bladder, so a rubber catheter will be used to remove urine and may be kept in place until time for pushing.
- Studies have shown that the mother has a greater chance of developing a fever if labor is slowed or prolonged after receiving the epidural, and it remains in place longer than 10 hours. Antibiotics will and can be administered. To decrease the chance of this occurrence, it is important that the mother be in good, active labor, be dilated at least 4 to 6 centimeters, and that the baby be in a favorable position before receiving an epidural.
- A small percentage of women will experience "hot spots," or partial numbing. This occurs when a small spot on the body where contractions are felt will not completely numb, or when half of the body (below the naval) will not numb. This problem can usually be corrected with changing the mother's position or re-administration of the epidural.

- Studies have shown that a small number of women will experience lower backache or tenderness at the injection site for weeks to months after the epidural.

Who can't receive an epidural?

- Women who have severe scoliosis at the epidural placement site or those women with scoliosis who have had Harrington implant (or Harrington rod) surgery, making the placement impossible.
- Women with a low platelet count. Your healthcare provider will order your blood work when you arrive at the hospital. If your blood count is extremely low, it will increase your chances of bleeding so that epidurals can't be used.
- Women who are allergic to the medications used in an epidural.
- Women who have had fusion of their discs in the lower back at the epidural placement site.

Local anesthesia

If you haven't received an epidural and you need perineal repair from tissue separation (tear) or from an episiotomy, you will be given an anesthetic medication at the site. This will numb the perineum so you won't feel any suturing.

When a Caesarean Birth Becomes Necessary

Reasons for Caesarean birth (C-birth):

- Fetal Distress
- CPD – cephalo-pelvic-disproportion
- Malpresentation—breech or shoulder presentation
- Prolapsed Cord
- Placenta Previa
- Abruptio Placentae

In the United States, approximately 27 percent of women deliver babies by C-births. This is a major surgery so your healthcare provider will discuss with you all the risks. You can decrease your risk of having a C-birth by maintaining an upright position for labor, by walking or moving your hips that helps line your baby up in your pelvis correctly. You can also decrease the chances of having a C-birth by delaying getting an epidural until you are in good, active labor, and have dilated at least 4 to 6 centimeters. This decreases the need to use Pitocin, which may cause fetal distress.

When writing your birth plan, include your wishes and desires just in case a C-birth is needed. Some of the options you may wish to discuss will be:

- Having your support person next to you during the surgery. (For emergencies, or with use of general anesthesia, this request may be limited.)

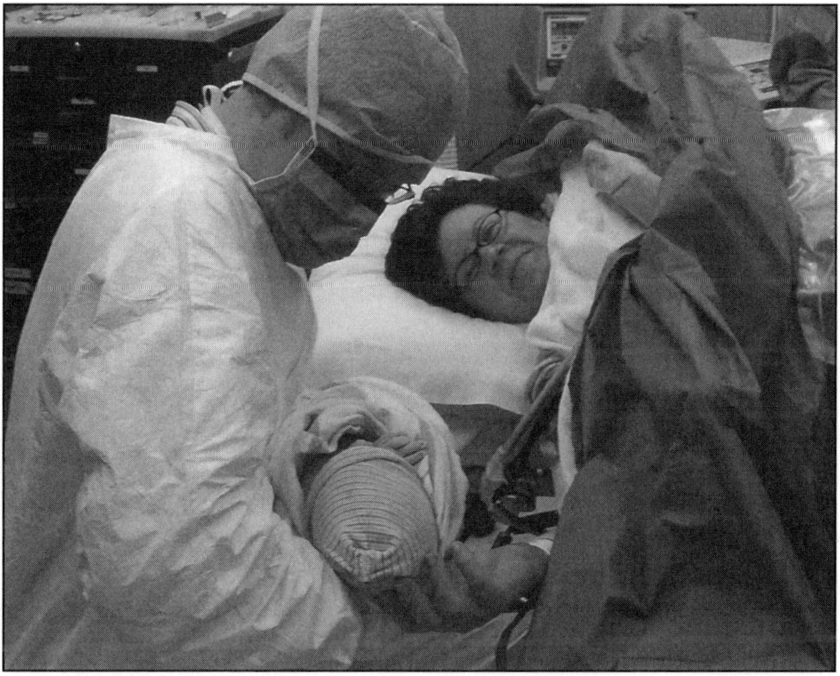

Support during a C-birth is important as shown with Ger holding his new daughter, Maeve, so Jennifer can touch and see her.

- If you think you would like to watch the actual birth, have the nurse bring in a mirror and tilt it at the head of the operating table.
- Have someone take pictures for you. I like pictures of the baby's head and shoulders coming out and the baby on your belly. The doctor usually holds the baby over the drape for you to see your little one. Many of my couples like these pictures in black and white.
- Have your support person stay close to the baby while she is getting examined under the warmer. Have the nurse bring the baby to you so you can see her, touch her, and talk to her.
- Request to breastfeed as soon as possible after delivery. This usually occurs in the recovery room.
- In the recovery room, keep your baby skin to skin.
- If your baby needs to go to the special care nursery, have your support person or your partner go with your baby. If you have a doula, have the doula stay with you.
- If, for whatever reason, general anesthesia is needed, and your partner or support person can't be in the room with you, ask the nurse to bring the baby to your partner or support person to hold while the doctors complete your surgery.

Recovery:

Your recovery from a C-birth will take longer than that of a vaginal birth. You will stay in the hospital one or possibly two days longer. You will need help with getting out of bed the first few times. You will need pain medications for several days up to several weeks. For the first 24 hours after surgery, your diet is usually limited to clear liquids or soft, bland foods. The day after surgery, your IV fluids will be discontinued and your bladder catheter will be removed. The nurses or lactation consultant will help you find comfortable positions for breastfeeding. Once you get home, your frequency of going up and down the stairs may be limited to once or twice a day since this increases pain and discomfort at the incision site.

Before you leave the hospital, or at your six weeks postpartum visit, be sure to discuss the possibility of having a vaginal birth for your next pregnancy. This is called a VBAC—vaginal birth after cesarean. Whether you can have a VBAC depends on the reasons for your initial C-birth.

Be sure to discuss your feelings about having the C-birth. Many women feel angry, disappointed, sad or a combination of all these feelings and more. Talking with a supportive person will help to validate your feelings. It can also help you sort out your feelings, which can be very complex and emotionally charged.

Remember:

- Education is important. Sign up for a childbirth education class early in your pregnancy.
- Understanding the labor process provides you with confidence to trust your body's ability.
- Encourage your partner to learn comfort measures, relaxation and breathing techniques in order to support you during birth.
- Consider hiring a certified doula.

CHAPTER FOUR

Postpartum

The Homecoming

Homecoming is an exciting time. You may have visualized this moment of bringing your baby home to a peaceful place where your new family can relax, bond, and settle into your new roles. This can more easily happen if you get yourself organized and set things in place. Before doing this, you need to examine your mindset for postpartum.

Many couples attend childbirth classes to learn about the birth process, but few couples prepare themselves as much for the postpartum period. After delivery, you will spend two to three days recovering in the hospital. You will learn how to care for your newborn, how to change diapers and bathe a baby, and given many tips on the challenges of breastfeeding, as well as entertaining visitors. On the day of discharge, the nurse will assist you with getting your things together, along with reviewing a list of last minute instructions. Then she will wheel you down to your car and make sure you have secured your baby in the car seat, and help to place all your items in the trunk. She'll smile, say goodbye, and wish you well as she closes your car door. The three of you drive off. Reality sets in.

From here, if you have a postpartum plan, things should continue to move smoothly. Sadly, most people don't realize how unprepared they are until they're in the middle of it. New parents can feel incredibly overwhelmed, stressed, sleep deprived, inadequately prepared and alone.

This is why evaluating your mindset for postpartum is just as important as thinking about your mindset for pregnancy and birth. You can use the blank pages in the back of this book, or simply use the below space to answer the following questions.

Your Mindset for Postpartum

1. Have you or your partner ever cared for a newborn?

   no

2. Who will be helping you the first few weeks after birth?

   Stafford. After 1-2 weeks, Grandmom;

3. Do you plan to attend newborn care classes? If yes, are you registered?

   Yes, Yes

4. Have you ever bathed a newborn?

   no

5. List four items you will need to bathe your baby:

   wash cloth

   simple soap

   baby bath tub

   a dirty baby

6. Are you planning to breastfeed your baby? If so, do you have a good support system?

   Yes, Yes

7. Write down two people/groups you could contact to obtain breastfeeding support. Look up phone numbers now and place them on your refrigerator door.

   Pedatric Assoc of RVA

   La Leche league

8. If you are planning to bottle feed, have you purchased bottles, appropriate size nipples, cleaning brushes or bottle liners? (Don't purchase large quantities of formula until after your baby is born.)

No

9. Whether breast or bottle feeding, how often does a newborn need to be fed?

2-3 hr / wheneve they hung

10. How will you be able to tell that your breastfeeding baby is getting adequate milk intake in a 24-hour period?

the output and gaining weight

11. Who will be helping with nighttime feedings? (mom, dad, grandparent, postpartum doula)

mom and dad

12. Are you using cloth or disposable diapers? (Don't purchase large quantities of newborn size.)

Cloth

13. Where do you plan for your baby to sleep? (bassinet, crib, co-sleeper, your bed)

crib in bedroom

14. How many hours on average do newborns sleep?

tbd

15. At what age do you think your newborn will sleep the entire night (from 8 p.m. to 6 a.m.)?

______

16. Crying is your baby's way of communicating. How many hours a day do normal, healthy newborns cry?

    ?, 1hr + spaced out; feed before crying

17. What is the earliest you can take your newborn outside the house?

    a couple days for newborn check up

18. While you are home on maternity leave, research support groups in your area. Below are a few types of groups that can be good sources of support. Spend a little time looking up information about what they offer and when they meet.

    Breastfeeding groups ______

    Stroller Strides ______

    New mother groups ______

    Baby and Me Yoga ______

    Postpartum depression groups ______

    Infant massage ______

19. How many weeks after the baby is born can you re-establish your routine exercise program?

    whatever Dr. says - 4-6 wks?

20. List 4 forms of exercise you like to do, either with or without your baby.

    Run, yoga, pilates, hiking/walking

    ______

    ______

    ______

21. Have you purchased the following items that mom may need at the house the first few weeks? (Check with your doctor about pain meds.)

    Motrin/Advil ____ Breast pads if breastfeeding ___
    Tylenol ____ Lanolin ointment ____
    Sanitary pads ____ Nursing Bras _____
    Tucks/hemorrhoid pads ____
    Notebook to record feedings/stools/voiding ____
    Snacks that can be eaten with one hand ____
    Bottled water or two large containers for water ____
    Reference books:
    One on breastfeeding, one on newborn care ____

22. Make a list of important phone numbers on an index card and place on your refrigerator door or next to your phone. Include: Your doctor's number, baby's doctor's number, emergency numbers including local poison control, all contact numbers for you and your partner.

23. In the blank pages of this book, or on a separate sheet of paper, write a list of household tasks you do on a regular basis and that will need to be done for the first four weeks postpartum (vacuum, dust, laundry, groceries).

24. In the blank pages of this book, or on a separate piece of paper, list the favorite foods that you and your partner love to eat so when your family and friends call to ask what they can prepare for you, you don't need to think; it's written down.

Great job on completing all the questions, including writing the list of items needed during the postpartum period. By doing these things early, you will make the homecoming transition move much smoother. It will also help you think about your mindset for the postpartum period; it helps you set realistic goals for yourself and your baby. Most women think they can still do it all—the cooking, cleaning, caring for her partner, family and now, this newest member. It can be very overwhelming, especially when combined with sleep deprivation. Writing down your postpartum plan and calling your family and friends to schedule help will eliminate much unneeded stress later.

Your Hospital Stay

On the hospital's postpartum unit, the nurses will check your vital signs (blood pressure, temperature, pulse), and will check your uterus. They massage the fundus (top of uterus) to make sure it is firm, and will ask about vaginal discharge (lochia), frequency of voiding and bowel movements, and will provide pain medication if requested. They will also provide some education concerning your health and your newborn's care. You can choose to have your baby "room-in" the entire time, which is great for bonding and learning about your baby's hunger and communication cues. Some mothers have their babies stay in their hospital room for the day and in the nursery at night. Some mothers want their babies to stay in the nursery all of the time except during feedings. Your doctor, midwife or one of their associates will visit each day. Your baby's pediatrician will also come by and answer questions, as well as tell you the baby's daily weight, and discuss any procedures ordered for your baby. Remember, you need to be informed of procedures done on you and your baby.

The following explains the general characteristics of your baby and some of the procedures performed on your baby.

The Newborn

The actual birth of your baby is a special time—greeting this new little person into your life, seeing the beautiful features of your baby's face, gazing into her eyes, making that special bond. Your life will never be the same, as it will be enhanced with love, joy and laughter, while at the same time understanding your responsibility, which is to raise your baby in a loving, nurturing environment and to teach her life skills and life-long values. All of this may seem overwhelming, but just remember, you have your child's lifetime in which to accomplish these things.

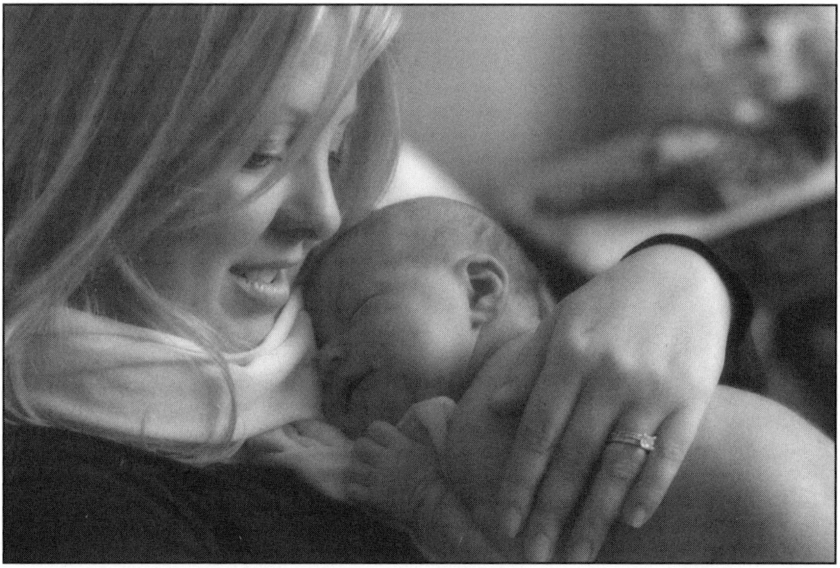

Heather snuggles with her newborn daughter, Pressley Shea.
Photo by Portraits by Jody.

Bonding

Bonding is a special time when the first exchanges of eye contact, tender touching, and soft talking between you and the baby occur. This early interaction helps lay the foundation for your parent-child relationship. This kind of bonding also occurs when your partner spends this special time with baby. If all goes well in labor and delivery, the first hours after birth is when bonding usually occurs. In some cases, such as a C-birth under general anesthesia, or if your baby requires emergency medical care and is taken to the intensive care unit, then this special bonding time can occur later.

During this bonding period, you and your baby will gaze at each other and your baby will sometimes begin to mirror some of your expressions. Many parents are amazed at how "smart" their babies are as well as how fast their babies begin to mimic their facial expressions. Besides feelings of excitement and deep love for your baby, you will feel surges of protectiveness and awe. These interactive moments are part of the attachment process, and both parents and baby benefit from this "falling in love" period.

In the first few weeks after birth, most of the bonding occurs without effort. You are taking in and processing the birth, beginning to understand the demands of caring for your newborn, such as how to function on very little sleep, and learning new skills for breastfeeding and baby care. The characteristics of your baby will change quickly over the first few weeks of life. Understanding these normal changes will decrease undue hours of worry, giving you more time to relax and enjoy your baby.

Characteristics of Your Newborn

Head:

Your baby's head may appear to be an odd shape immediately at birth. This is called "molding" and is due to the baby's skull bones overlapping so that the head will fit through the birth canal. Usually within 24 to 48 hours, the misshapened head will return to normal.

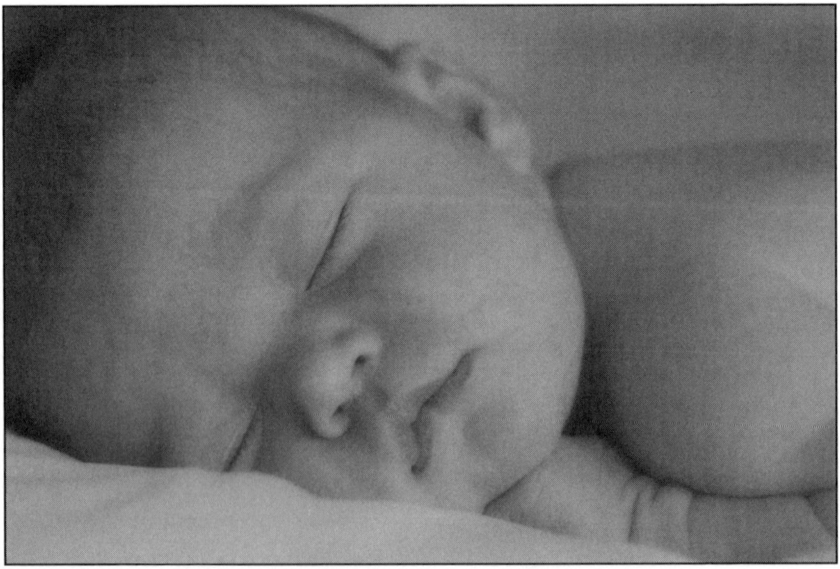

Pressley sleeps on her mother's chest. ***Remember: Back to sleep when in crib.*** *Photo by Portraits by Jody.*

If forceps or a vacuum extractor are used to assist in the birth, you may notice bruising on the top or sides of the head. This usually resolves within the first few days of life. Occasionally, a baby may develop a large "goose egg," or knot, on the top of the head off to one side. This is called a cephalohematoma which is caused by bleeding underneath the skin outside the skull. While this may take months to resolve, it causes no harm, and your baby's pediatrician will keep a close eye on it until it is resolved.

Eyes:

At birth, the eyelids can be puffy and if you look closely, you may notice fine eye lashes and eye brows. Most babies have blue, slate blue or brown eyes. The true color appears between 6 to 12 months. Due to the shape and puffiness, the eyes may appear crossed. When your baby learns to focus, her eyes may occasionally cross. If you notice that your baby's eyes always turn inward, or if you have a family history of strabismus (lazy eye), tell your baby's healthcare provider. An eye exam by a pediatric ophthalmologist will be necessary in the first few months of life.

You may notice a small red hemorrhage on the conjunctiva (white part of the eye). This is due from the pressure of birth, causing no visual problems and will resolve over several days without treatment.

Clogged tear ducts are common during the first few months of life. You may notice a discharge in one or both eyes. Call your baby's healthcare provider for eye drops and instructions for massaging the tear duct. Many mothers squirt a little breast milk onto each eye and gently rub it in.

Nose:

The nose may appear flat or misshapened at birth. This will correct itself the first week of life. Most parents notice that the baby's nose will sound "stuffy" a few days to weeks after birth. This can cause sleeping and eating issues since babies are nose breathers. One reason is that the baby may have had "spit up" and a small amount of milk came up through the nose. If all the milk doesn't come out, it causes a stuffy sound when the baby breathes. Another common reason, especially if your baby is born during the winter months, is that the air in your house may be too dry due to the heating system. The body tries to correct the problem by producing mucus for moisture. The easiest way is to turn down the thermostat in the house to between 68° and 70° F, and add moisture by using a room humidifier. Ask your baby's healthcare provider about using children's saline nasal spray.

Mouth:

Your baby's lips are very sensitive, and after 2 to 3 weeks of breastfeeding, a small callous may form on the upper lip. This can be gently peeled off. If you ever notice any white patches on the inside of the mouth, on the cheeks, tongue or gums, you need to call the baby's healthcare provider. This is a common yeast condition known as thrush. If you are breastfeeding, both mother and baby need to be treated at the same time.

Ears:

Shape of the ears usually looks like someone in the family. In many states, it is mandatory that a newborn hearing screening be done before leaving the hospital. Be sure to tell the baby's healthcare provider of any family history of congenital deafness.

Neck:

Most babies appear as if they don't have a neck. Due to weak neck muscles, it is important to support the baby's head at all times. Soon your baby will be able to lift her head, increasing neck muscle strength. When bathing, be sure to wash and dry the creasing of the neck. Sweat and spit up can collect in the creases, causing skin redness and irritation, as well as a sour, yeasty smell.

Chest:

Your baby may have enlarged breasts, one or both, regardless of gender. This is caused by mother's hormones the baby received in utero. This resolves by itself in the first few weeks.

You may notice a bony "knot" slightly below the breast bone, center of the chest. This is the very lower tip of the breast bone. As the child grows, the developing chest muscles will cover it.

Abdomen:

Babies have poor abdominal muscles, which gives the appearance of a "potbelly," especially after eating. By age 2 to 3 years, the abdominal muscles get stronger and this "potbelly" appearance fades.

The umbilical cord stump needs to be treated like a scab. The sooner it dries up, the sooner it will fall off. Some healthcare providers suggest wiping the cord with rubbing alcohol once a day, while others suggest keeping it totally dry. It usually takes anywhere from 1 to 3 weeks to fall off. Occasionally, after the cord has fallen off, a small piece of cord tissue remains in the center of the umbilicus. This tissue looks yellowish and whitish, and may produce a pinkish brown discharge on the diaper or t-shirt. This is known as a granuloma. The baby's healthcare provider will simply treat this in the office with an application of silver nitrate, which causes it to dry up and disappear.

Genitals:

Both male and female genitals are swollen at birth due to the mother's hormones received in utero. In females, the mother's hormones are also responsible for the whitish vaginal mucus discharge you may see. For some girl babies, at 10 to 14 days of life, you may see pseudo-menstruation, or a "false period"; vaginal discharge will turn a pinkish, bloody color. It may last anywhere from one diaper change up to 2 days. It may seem strange or alarming, but it is perfectly normal.

In males, the scrotum can appear swollen and fluid, known as a hydrocele, can collect around one or both testicles. This is usually benign and will be followed by the baby's healthcare provider.

By the time of birth, most parents have made the decision to circumcise or not. Check out the American Academy of Pediatrics website at www.AAP.org for the pros and cons of this procedure.

Circumcision for your son is a personal decision. This common surgical procedure is done by the ob/gyn or the family practice doctor on the second day of life. Some doctors numb the penis before cutting the foreskin, others still don't. Be sure to ask that they do numb the area. In my area (Richmond, VA), many pediatric urologists are performing the circumcision procedure in their office within the first month of life. Inquire about a pediatric urologist in your area.

Extremities:

Many parents worry about the appearance of the baby's feet and legs. Some of the odd positions are just that, positional, and will correct themselves with tincture of time. Baby's legs may appear bowed or the feet turned in, or upward, too far. The two bones in the lower leg will straighten out by age 2 to 3 years. Feet straighten out quickly with simple stretching exercises.

Skin:

At birth, your baby may be covered with vernix, a white waxy, cheese-like, substance that protects your baby's skin as he lives in the amniotic fluid throughout your pregnancy. The amount of vernix present at birth depends on the week of gestation. Babies born past the due date usually have very little vernix on the body except in the folds and creases of his skin.

You may notice in the first days of life that your baby's skin might have a "flea bite" looking rash that comes and goes and can be found anywhere on the body. This benign rash will usually last 1 to 2 weeks. The cause of this is unknown.

You may also notice the little whiteheads found on the baby's face and nose. These are called *milia* and will disappear without treatment in several weeks. The next facial rash you will see is "newborn acne." This appears around 4 weeks of life and will last about 4 weeks. It looks like acne and appears on the face and head, but never below the nipple line. Some days it looks worse than others, but the skin will eventually become completely clear. The severity of baby acne does not predict the amount of adolescent acne.

The Measurements and What They Mean

Weight:

All babies are weighed at birth. It is exciting to get the "number." Babies can lose up to 8 percent of their birth weight during the first week of life and will regain it all back, plus more, by the end of the second week. Most babies, especially breastfeeding babies, will gain ½ to 1 ½ oz. per day, which is 1 to 2 pounds per month. The average baby will double its birth weight between 4 to 6 months and triple it by one year. Your baby's weight will be one of the measurements that will be graphed on a standardized scale at your baby's healthcare provider's office. This aids the healthcare provider in watching for appropriate growth. The healthcare provider will give your child's percentage at each visit. Your baby's weight is compared to the weights of 100 other same sex babies of the same age. For example, a male baby in the 75th percentile for weight at 2 months of age means that he weighs more than 75 out of 100 male babies at the same age.

NOTE: If your breastfeeding baby is a slow gainer, be sure the healthcare provider is using the graph for breastfeeding infants. Breastfeeding babies can gain at a slower rate and be perfectly healthy.

Height:

This measurement will be done at birth and again at each well baby checkup. Don't get upset if it appears your baby isn't growing in length like you think she should. Stretching the legs out can be difficult the first few weeks. By 9 months, your baby's height will be at a more normal percentage for your family history. The height will be another measurement plotted on the standardized growth chart.

Head Circumference:

Your baby's head will be measured at birth and then at every routine well baby checkup. This measurement will also be plotted and will be monitored to ensure normal head growth.

All three measurements—weight, height, and head circumference—will be a guide to your baby's normal growth and development. These will each be assessed at every well baby checkup. Additional information collected during routine visits is the daily number of wet diapers and number of stools. This information also aids in determining that your baby is thriving.

Stools:

Shortly after birth, your baby will pass the first stool called meconium. It is very thick, black and sticky. As the baby increases protein feedings, especially with breast milk feedings, the quicker the baby will pass the entire meconium stool. Several days of brownish-green stools follow, which then lead to yellow, seedy-looking stools. The number of stools a baby has on a daily basis is also important. The more breast milk the baby gets, the more stools he will pass.

As for the formula-fed baby, the amount of milk the baby is drinking can easily be measured. For the breastfed baby, the

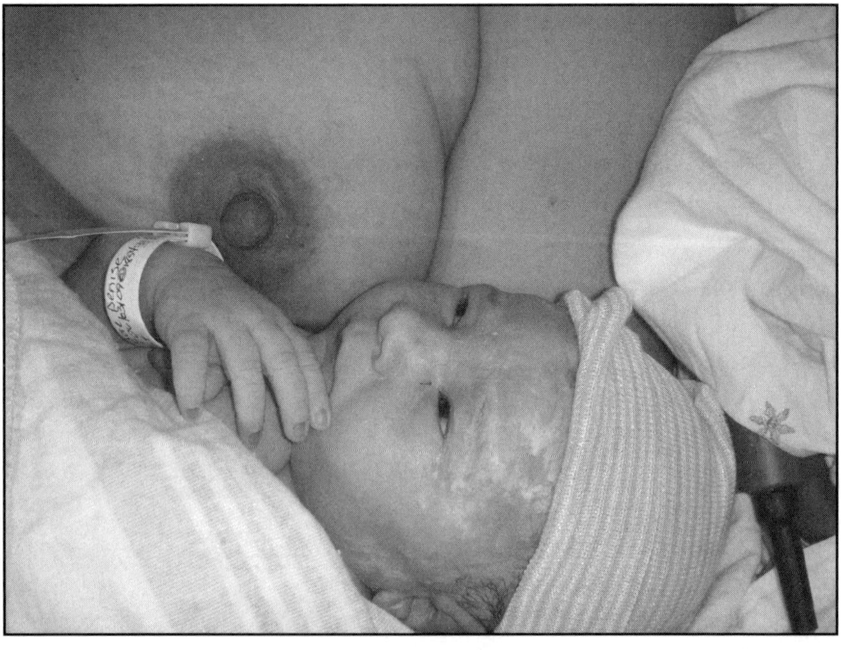

Just minutes old, Simone is alert and ready to nurse.

number of stools per day is the guide for adequate intake of breast milk. Three or more yellow-seedy stools everyday is ideal. Some babies have a small yellow stool with every feeding; this is also normal.

Voiding:

Babies urinate small amounts and with the absorption of disposable diapers today, the quantity can sometimes be difficult to determine. If the number of voidings is in question, place a tissue in the diaper; if the tissue is wet, your baby has voided. This is only important the first week at home. After the milk intake is adequate, babies will void 6 to 12, or more, times a day.

Sleep:

During the immediate newborn period your baby will sleep 12-20 hours her first day of life as she acclimates to her new environment. The first night at home, your baby may stay awake and be fussy for 4-6 hours straight. The second night is usually much better. This begins the sleep deprivation period. During this time, if your baby is sleeping for 4-6 hour periods at one time, it is important to wake her at least every 3 hours to feed until your milk supply is well established and she has gained back to her birth weight and beyond. As the first week or two passes, her sleeping periods will be short but frequent. It's common for her to awaken every 1 ½ -3 hours for feedings, stay alert for a few minutes, then back to sleep. Her sleep pattern will be unpredictable, so it is important for you to sleep when she sleeps. As she grows and gains weight, she will be able to go longer periods of time between feedings and will be able to stay awake for longer stretches. This is when she will become more social.

Postpartum for Mom

Many of your needs will be the same as your baby's—eating, sleeping, playing, grooming, etc.

Eating:

It is important for you to keep your energy level high and to feed your body healthy foods to aid in healing. You will be eating fruits, vegetables, proteins and grains. Eat a variety of foods. If you are breastfeeding, remember that some foods that give you gas may also give your baby gas.

Rest/Sleep:

The first few weeks you are home, you will need to rest or sleep every time the baby sleeps. Your baby may have many fussy nights and not have slept much at night. This means you will not have slept either. You need your rest. Sleep deprivation is very hard to handle and is unhealthy for the mind and body. If you feel you can't sleep during the day because you need to watch the baby, get someone to help you.

Play:

Once the first few weeks have passed and you are feeling like you have a "little" pattern, you may wish to meet a friend for lunch or go to the mall with a friend. Life does go on with a baby. Getting out will feed your emotional side. The four walls of your house can start to feel as if they are closing in on you if you don't get out.

Grooming:

You will find that daily showers just make you feel better. The first weeks after birth your hormones are "getting back to normal," you may notice night sweats—this is common. Showering feels great. If you are home alone and worry about the baby, put her in her infant car seat and take her in the bathroom with you. If you have extra help to watch the baby, take a long, relaxing shower. You will also feel better if by noon you have simply gotten dressed, brushed your teeth and combed your hair. You may laugh when you read that sentence, thinking you'll have plenty of time for those kinds of things. In reality, you may chuckle (or maybe you won't find it so funny at all!) when the day comes that you haven't gotten dressed or brushed your teeth before 4:00 in the afternoon.

The first few weeks after birth you may notice the following changes in your body. All are normal and will go away without any medical treatment. These temporary changes are:

- Night sweats
- Hot flashes
- Hair loss
- Hemorrhoids
- Sleep deprivation
- Breast pain
- After birth pains

If you notice any of the following warning signs, seek medical attention immediately:

- Increase in vaginal bleeding (called lochia) after first week. The amount of lochia should decrease in amount and the color should change from bright red to brownish-pink. If you notice clots bigger than a quarter or a foul-smelling odor, call immediately—this could mean a hemorrhage or an infection.
- Fever. Even a low-grade fever—a temperature over 100 degrees orally—can mean an infection.
- Redness or pain in the breast. If you notice one red spot on one breast, it's probably a clogged milk duct. But if your entire breast is red, painful, hot, this is more serious and could be signs of mastitis, an infection of the breast tissue.
- Severe or persistent pain or tenderness in your leg, usually the calf area, or if one leg is more swollen than the other.

- Severe or persistent headaches, with or without double vision, blurring, or dimming of vision, or flashing spots or lights.
- Severe or persistent pain anywhere in your abdomen or pelvis, or if your afterbirth pains are getting worse instead of better.
- Beyond the first week, any redness, swelling or discharge at the incision site from your C-birth needs to be reported. This is also true of continuous, severe pain in the vaginal and rectal area due to episiotomy pain, stitches or hemorrhoids.
- Burning or painful urination—also any increase, or frequency, or urgency to void.
- Persistent vomiting.
- Extreme sadness or despair, or having delusions, or thoughts of harming yourself or your baby.

Postpartum Depression

I would like to spend a little more time here on the seriousness of postpartum depression. It is a medical condition that will get worse if you do not get help.

If you are experiencing sadness, despair, find yourself crying for days; if you can't care for yourself or your baby; if you are having delusions, visions, or thoughts of harming yourself or your baby, you are experiencing postpartum depression.

This condition may not occur immediately. It might take days, weeks or months before symptoms occur. ***You need to get help.*** Call your healthcare provider. He or she can prescribe medications or give you a name of a psychiatrist or therapist who specializes in postpartum depression. You may not need medication, but talking with a therapist can help greatly. If you do need medication, do not worry about having to stop breastfeeding because of it, as there are many medications that can be safely used while breastfeeding. You may also find you need extra help with the baby or housework from a postpartum doula, friend or family member.

The postpartum period is an exciting and tiring time. While all the physical and emotional changes are occurring to mothers, dads and partners are also experiencing emotional changes. So much attention is focused on the mother, we often forget that dads and partners need support also. In most of the couples I work with, the dads and partners are present during the birth, providing back pressure, massage, slow dancing, providing support and encouragement throughout labor and delivery. They usually stay at the hospital for the next two days, helping with night feedings, learning how to change diapers and provide care for the baby, worrying about mom's and baby's health and well-being and taking in the overwhelming event of becoming a parent. Sometimes there are worries about financial issues, providing for the family, and living up to real or imagined expectations. Getting extra help will also allow your partner to get rest, or will allow the opportunity to run errands or get things done outside the home. Supporting each other will help you both with a smoother transition into parenthood.

Remember:

- Mindset of postpartum—planning ahead will eliminate many hours of undue stress.
- Make a list of household tasks that will need to be done—set up extra help now.
- List your favorite foods—welcome gifts of homemade "comfort" foods and then enjoy.
- Get two resource books—one on breastfeeding and one on general baby care.
- Ask for, and get help when you need it! If you are in doubt about whether you need help, ask for help. There is no such thing as too much support.
- Relax!! Take a deep breath. Don't forget to take care of yourself.

CHAPTER FIVE
Parenthood

This is the transition in life that defines the true meaning of the word responsibility. No more hopping into the car at the last minute going to a movie or out to eat. No more sleeping in until 10 a.m. after partying late into the early hours of the morning. No more spending your spare money on toys like electronic equipment without strict budgeting first. Most new parents are so focused on their precious baby, those things mentioned above take second place. This is a time in your life when this new life is totally dependent on you for love, food, warmth and care. Your new baby needs to be provided for physically, emotionally, and spiritually. As a parent, you will provide your child with all these things. You will also teach your child life lessons...sharing your gifts and talents, teaching values to help this child become a well-adjusted, responsible, educated adult who will pass down the same values to his/her children as well as share with the world their gifts and talents. Your child may grow up to be a world leader, famous author, respected doctor or lawyer, teacher, gold medal Olympian...the list is endless. It all starts with providing this child with a safe place to live and grow, opportunities to learn and excel with patience and encouragement along the entire way. You are your child's advocate and cheerleader. You are also your child's guide through the good times and the difficult ones. This means providing discipline with love. You are not your child's best friend…that's why you hold the proud title of Mom or Dad.

What is your mindset on becoming a parent? Again, I have a list of questions to get you thinking of what you want for your child. Remember, having a positive picture of what you want will set these thoughts in action and your dreams can come true.

Your Mindset on Becoming a Parent

1 List three feelings you have about becoming a parent.

a. ______________________________

b. ______________________________

c. ______________________________

2. Name three characteristics/assets, you have that will make you a good parent.

a. ______________________________

b. ______________________________

c. ______________________________

3. Write three characteristics/assets your partner has that will make him/her a good parent.

a. ______________________________

b. ______________________________

c. ______________________________

4. What are two family traditions you would like to continue?

a. ______________________________

b. ______________________________

5. Name five things you would like to do with your children/family before your children turn 18 years of age.

a. ______________________________

b. ______________________________

c. ______________________________

d. ______________________________

e. ______________________________

6. What dreams do you have for your baby?
   a. ______________________________
   b. ______________________________
   c. ______________________________

7. Think of one or two pictures you wish you had of your childhood (pictures with your dad playing ball in the yard, or helping your mom bake cookies at Christmas). Make wonderful memories with your children. What are two of your favorite pictures of yourself as a child?
   a. ______________________________
   b. ______________________________

Along with all the good times, there will be times of exhaustion, frustration, disappointment, and feelings of wanting to give up. This is when you need to remember, "I can handle it," regardless of what is placed in front of you. It may be a time to take a break. These times will happen. Go sit quietly by the water or an open field—some place where you are alone and able to think clearly. As you sit and reflect, don't focus on the things that are going wrong, but on the things you are doing right. What have you accomplished in life up to this point? Have a job? Career? Good relationship with your partner, parents and friends? Beautiful family? Good health? Friends? Success? Think of these things and think of the beauty surrounding you… the sun, the trees, the flowers, the sky, birds, butterflies, the warmth of the sun on your skin, or the breeze through your hair.

If you find yourself in a poor relationship with your partner or family, get help to resolve the issues. If you were wrong, admit it, and say you are sorry. Life is too short to miss one day of a family's love and the feeling of peace in your heart that comes when you know things are right between you and those you love.

The support you received or provided during your birth journey will always be remembered and appreciated. During the quiet moments of parenthood, be sure to express your gratitude and appreciation to your partner for this gift of love and support. I have been so blessed over the past fifteen years to be invited to attend over 160 births. I feel very privileged to have been with new mothers and fathers and witnessed the births of their beautiful babies. Several of these new parents wish to share their birth experiences with you.

BIRTH STORIES

This section contains birth stories from mothers and fathers whom I had the privilege of meeting, either in my Lamaze class or as being their doula. These are the birth stories of these families written in the words of either the mother or father of the newborn baby. I have not changed the substance of any of these stories. I thank each and every one of them for allowing their stories to be shared here.

Austin's Birth Story

I was due with my second child, a daughter, in early August. My son was almost two and I was more than ready to have this little girl out of my belly. This second pregnancy had been much more uncomfortable (ok, painful) on my body; just aches and pains on my joints and my back. But just like with my first pregnancy, my body wasn't budging…even on the due date. So, I went over my due date by about a week, and then, because of a combination of doctor policies and my doctor going on vacation, I was basically forced to choose an induction for Friday morning of that week. While I definitely didn't want to be induced, I was also glad to know that FINALLY this baby would be here.

With my first, my son, I had all intentions of "going natural" with no drugs, but after some Pitocin that I had to take because I wasn't progressing, I begged for the epidural. This time, I was going to try again, and had the help of not only my husband, but also my aunt Kathy, a trained doula.

The doctor broke my water early that morning. (I think "icky" is the proper term for how that feels.) After that, we began our cycle of trying to get the labor going on its own: lots of walking while I was allowed off the monitor and hot towels on my boobs while I was in bed on the monitor. Surely enough, contractions started coming. They got to the point that I had to stop walking and talking when one came. It was working and without Pitocin! Things progressed rather quickly and soon enough I was using the tub that was, THANKFULLY, in my room. At first, it was a great relief, but then the contractions got so strong that even the water didn't seem to be helping… plus it was time to be monitored again. (While my nurse did all she could to support my wishes, sometimes hospital policy prevailed.) Then came what I think was the hardest, most annoying, and most painful part of labor for me: moving. After I was at about 7 cm, every little move I tried to make—from one position to another—brought on a contraction.

So I finally made it from the tub to the birthing ball at the foot of the bed. This was the point when I started getting scared. I had never done this before—this was pain and nausea like I had never felt. I think half of the battle was my doubt in my decision: "Should I have taken the epidural while I could have? What have I done? Can I actually do this? I'm stuck now. There's no going back." There were so many thoughts running through my head. It was very emotional for me and I just remember being terrified.

Then it was time for me to move to the bed. At this point, I was in a really dark place of pain. I don't remember (thankfully!) exactly how I felt, but I remember not being able to speak or move and just thinking I would pass out. I also remember *screaming* at the nurse when she told me she wanted to "check" me while I was having a contraction.

Then, all of a sudden the nurse told me, "Ok, next time we're going to push."

What?!? I thought in disbelief, but it was time!

So the first couple of pushes were probably heard out in the parking lot (and the windows were closed). I don't remember the pain, just the need to scream. Then I guess I was doing pretty well because they made me take a little break so the doctor could get there in time to deliver the baby. The doctor arrived and heard one of my screaming pushes, and as mad as I was at her at that moment, she did give me some good advice. She told me to take all the energy I was putting into my screaming and just push. So I did some "silent" pushes... just a couple, actually... and Austin was out. I was definitely blessed to have a rather short labor (less than 6 hours) and very little pushing (probably less than 20 minutes).

So she was out, and I was simply in disbelief that I had just done that.

What enjoyment. I held my little girl and she smiled at me and nursed FOREVER. She was finally here!

Then, of course, it was time for her checkup and bath... and mine, too. I was almost giddy as I realized I could stand up, walk across the room, and shower myself. I couldn't stop smiling. When I was all clean and dressed, in came a wheelchair to take me to my recovery room. I gladly declined sitting down on my bum, and walked myself in my fuzzy slippers down to my room.

I spent the next few days and weeks getting into the swing of two children, finding it easier than I had thought it would be. My son was surprisingly patient and understanding. I also had the support of many women bringing meals, which was such a blessing.

Looking back on it the next few days, I was still unsure of my decision to go without the epidural. The pain stayed fresh for me a bit too long. But here I sit, pregnant once more, and even though I vowed never to do natural birth again, I am definitely wanting to go without drugs this time!

Father's view:

Our second child, Austin, has been strong-willed from the beginning and refused to come out until we decided to induce by breaking Stephanie's water. Once we did this, the birth flowed perfectly. Stephanie had decided to try to go natural for as long as possible but was not against an epidural if she felt it was needed. Having Kathy there for guidance and support throughout the

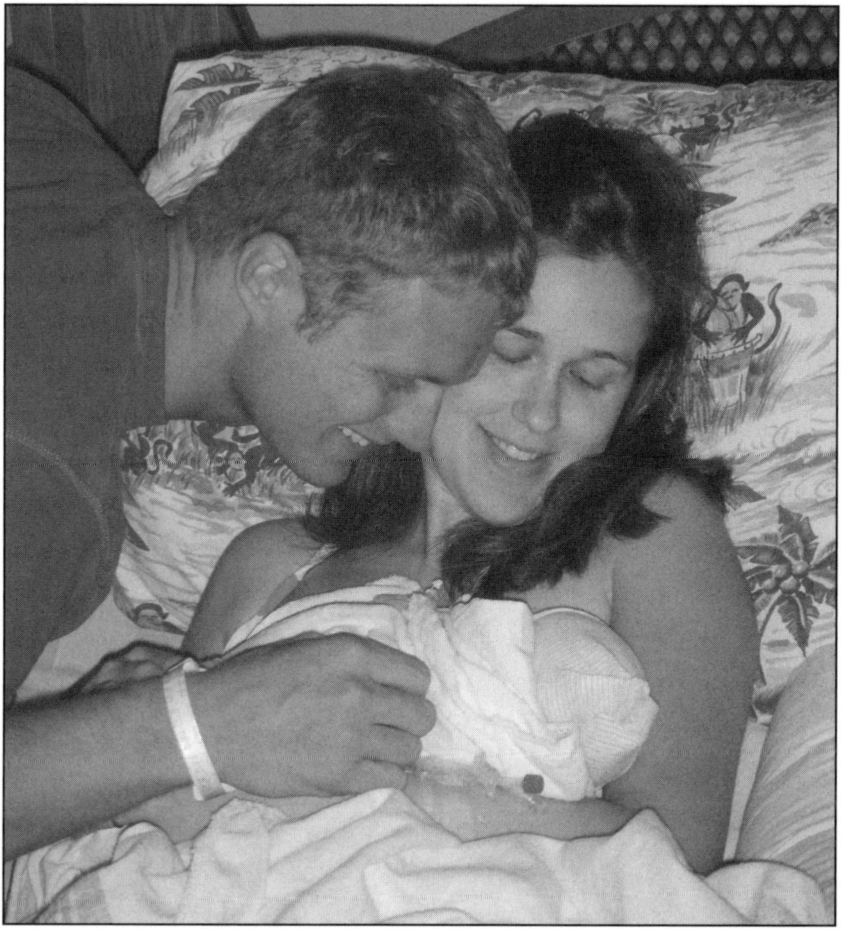

Michael and Stephanie gaze at their second child, first daughter, Austin Grace.

birth was crucial to her being able to birth naturally. We used a variety of means to do this, from walking, to sitting on the ball, to baths, and they all helped us get one step further. When it was time to push, Stephanie was ready and Austin came out quickly and fully alert. She immediately looked into our eyes and with her expression acknowledged us as her parents. From start to finish, it was a wonderful experience.

Baby Ellie's Birth Story – Baby #3 for Stephanie and Michael

The nine months of my third pregnancy seemed to fly by. I guess it was a combination of busy schedules and keeping up with two other children. Before I knew it, I was at the point where I didn't think my stomach could stretch any larger. The baby went overdue, which didn't surprise me, and as much as I envisioned having a quick labor that started on its own at home, I had to schedule an induction at 41 weeks. Knowing which day I would go into labor, as opposed to just being surprised, did make me nervous. I had done one birth with an epidural and one without. I was certainly hoping to go without again, but I just couldn't get my mind around the thought because I really couldn't remember exactly how it felt the last time.

Induction day came, and we arrived fashionably late after I dined on my breakfast that I wasn't "supposed" to have. It wasn't how I had planned on starting my labor, but it was finally here and I could stop worrying about when baby would come! I had a great nurse and my doula was there from the start, along with my husband. My mood was cheerful and chatty as I just wanted to get things going.

Just like baby #2, all the doctor had to do was break my water, and after a LOT of walking (hours!), contractions started. My legs finally got tired, so after numerous walks on each of my 40 minutes off the monitor, I decided to retire to the room. I did a little time on the ball and in the rocking chair, and then decided to take advantage of the shower, my favorite place!

I had labored in a tub for some of my last birth and I actually prefer the shower to the tub; I like how I could use hot water with a lot of pressure from the sprayer on my back and belly. I remember asking if I could just stay in there the whole time, birth and all!

After the shower, I got into bed, chilled from the labor and being wet. I labored sitting up for a while and got tired, so then moved to my side, where the contractions worsened tremendously… this was the first time I asked for the epidural because

I was discouraged to find out that I was still only 7 cm. But my husband and doula convinced me to try another position, and wow—what a difference that made. I then labored sitting up, almost in "Indian style," as I leaned over on my husband for quite awhile. I was encouraged to make it to 9 cm. I thought, Just a couple more contractions and I'm pushing this baby out!

I was wrong…very wrong. I think I stayed at 9 cm for about two hours with no changes; it was discouraging. We think the baby's head was turned in a way that didn't let her drop down. I tried laboring on my hands and knees and with the squat bar, but I couldn't manage the pain in those positions. I was tired and we had all decided it was time for an epidural.

So, right as I was sitting up to get in place for the needle, I uncontrollably started pushing. It was a sensation I had never felt, even with the last baby. I couldn't stop myself. Baby Ellie was born about 30 seconds later. Luckily, my doctor was in the room next door and got there in time to catch the baby… and luckily, the anesthesiologist was finishing up in another room and didn't make it!

Baby Ellie was finally here. I remember holding onto her so tightly, meanwhile being completely overwhelmed with emotions. It had been quite a roller coaster of emotions… for days really. And to have this labor take about four hours longer than my previous one was just unexpected. But baby was here, and that was all that mattered.

There were three main things that I came away with from this pregnancy, labor, and birth:

1.) Every pregnancy, labor, birth, and baby is different. There is no need wasting energy worrying about any of them based on past experiences because each is a new experience. This goes for different babies from the same mom as well as babies from different moms. While it is fun to compare birth stories, each person has their own for each child and everyone has a different pain threshold and way of describing their experiences. It is absolutely crazy to be discouraged by another's labor sounding easier than yours.
2.) Changing labor positions can do a lot!

3.) Really follow the doctor's instructions about not doing steps, lifting, or driving when you get home. I overdid it after baby #2, thinking, I handled natural childbirth, I can do it all, and ended up feeling horrible for weeks. This time I was good to myself, moved slowly, and acknowledged that my body had been through an awful lot. It paid off with a much quicker recovery so far!

By the way, it's been a week since the birth as I write this, and I've already forgotten the pains of labor; I just remember little moments of what I did, and then holding her as soon as she was born.

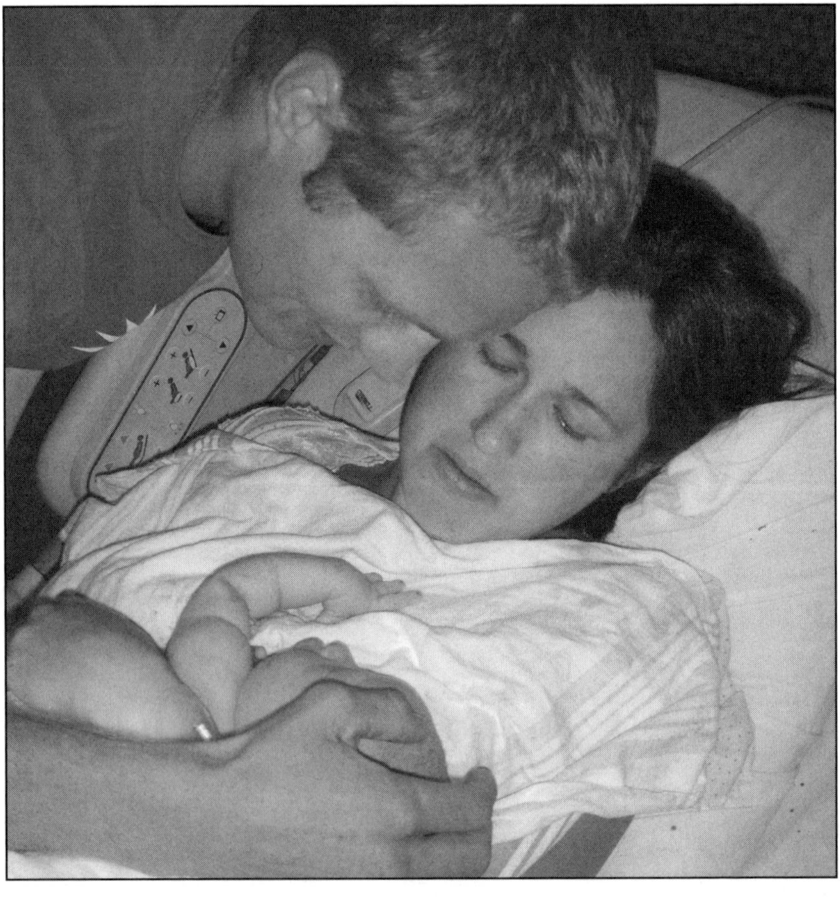

Michael and Stephanie welcome another daughter, Ellie Abigail.

Wyatt's Birth Story

A week before my due date, our doctor ordered an ultrasound, thinking our baby was going to be really big. The test came back that it was small (at 6.2 lb). The head looked great, the legs looked great, but the stomach was measuring small. Immediately, there was talk of induction and we were given two dates to choose from—Monday or Wednesday (we had the ultrasound on a Friday, which was one week and one day before my due date). I was surprised at how calm Jeff and I were—asking questions to understand why, and whether we could postpone the induction. Our doctor was really awesome. She gave us loads of information and even said that the test could be wrong—human error in measuring. We asked to get a second ultrasound to re-measure and hopefully avoid being induced.

I tried to stay positive and calm, but in my yoga class the next day, when we were going around to share stories, I totally broke down crying. I could barely put it into words, but all I knew was it just didn't feel right and I had really wanted the baby to tell my body "when" it needed to come, not let Pitocin tell me, unless it was truly necessary! I left yoga after a fabulous hour and a half of stretching, calmness and meditation and thought—let's see if we can beat this test on Monday. Best way to do that, I thought, was with hormone-laden food that's keeping America obese. McDonald's, here we come! It felt so wrong after a yoga class and so comforting at the same time!

So, I munched all weekend, which I doubt really made a difference, but when we had the ultrasound on Monday, the baby came back at 6 lb 10 oz! We were in the clear! However, my nurse practitioner didn't realize the doctor had said if the baby measures bigger we could cancel. So she kind of pushed for the induction saying it was great and by Wednesday I'd have a baby! Our doctor wasn't in the office that day, and instead of discussing it with the nurse practitioner, I just wrote to the doctor who responded that it was ok to cancel. Yay! Baby and I were on our way to letting him or her (since we didn't know the gender at that point) tell us when he would be ready for the world.

Later that week, Thursday, and one day after my "almost induction day," I woke up and just felt so tired. I was planning to go to Lewis Ginter Botanical Gardens and walk around, then run some errands. My body let me know that none of that was happening. So I relaxed, watched some TV and finished some notes I was writing, ate a HUGE meal around 2:30 and napped on and off.

At 5:00, I went upstairs and my water broke. I wasn't sure that's what it was, so I texted my husband, who I knew was in a meeting, and wrote: *I think my water just broke, can you call me when you get a chance?* I felt really calm and kind of excited. A few minutes later the phone rang, he thought it was hilarious that I texted him and said, "You should have just called!" Apparently he was on a conference call and put it on mute when he got my text so he could call me back. He said he heard in the background: "Jeff? Jeff? Oh...I wonder if he's on the phone with his wife." Which he was!

I told Jeff it wasn't like a gush of water but more of a pulsing—but each time it was like wetting my pants. He responded, "I think that means it's coming from high up, not low."

I was surprised. "How did you remember that from class?!" Then I remembered that Kathy had said the class was for the guys to remember everything since our brains would just kind of turn off when it was time for the baby! We were both very calm and excited. I called the doctor who was on call and we took our time. An hour and a half later we were at the hospital. By that time, the contractions were coming a lot closer together and were stronger. But I could still talk and joke a bit.

Upstairs, once I was in the room, dressed and had made it through all the millions of questions they asked, the contractions were about three and four minutes apart and were sharp! My L&D nurse was AWESOME. She read our birth plan and told us to "speak up about it" when the doctor came in and that "we didn't hear that from her." Again, since my "panties were off," it felt amazing to be empowered by another woman about my childbirth experience. The doctor on call came around 9:00 p.m. and said I had a long way to go and that I probably wouldn't deliver until the next day when our doctor was back on duty. So, he kind of wiped his hands clean of me, saying if the baby didn't come by morning, "your doctor and I can discuss Pitocin and next steps."

Whatever.

We were free to labor as we pleased from that point on.

The nurse told me about the pain killers and epidural, but said she would only tell me about it once because I wanted to labor as long as possible naturally. "I won't talk about them again. You will have to ask me if you want them, because I don't want you to think I'm saying you can't do this." Wow. I was floored and really amazed.

Jeff and I labored naturally for eight hours in the hospital until about 2:00 a.m. We used all of Kathy's techniques. I used my birth ball. I hopped in the shower, but not for long because I just went down on my knees in pain each time. I held onto Jeff; we did the "slow dance." I held onto him for dear life, thinking I might break his back, but I knew I couldn't walk or stand without him. I chanted through my contractions. I used my yoga breathing and on the exhaling would "OM" and make my voice go a bit deeper with each exhale, which made my shoulders drop, and Jeff said he could see and feel my body relax more. Kathy would have been so proud of him. Just so incredibly proud!!! He never left my side. He was there constantly reassuring me. With each contraction, just when my mind was telling me there was no way I'd live through this one, he would be saying "you're halfway there," and then the contraction would subside and I'd know I could make it. The labor was 50 percent me and 50 percent Jeff. I could not have done it without him. He was my rock, my love, my support, my empowerment, my true other half, and the literal strength that held me up.

I also threw up three times from the pain. Finally, when it was just cutting through me and I felt sick again and as if I were about to pass out, I asked for the narcotics. I'm so anti-medicine, but I did go in with an open mind. My goal was to try to go as long as I could naturally, but not to rule anything out. I went eight hours, and, as I told our doctor the next morning, before I took the narcotics, I thought I was going to see Heaven several times (and not in a good way) from all the pain.

I really am anti-medicine and I've never done any drugs. But man!! Now I know why people do!! They brought some type of narcotic and I felt GREAT! I felt like I was floating. But soon enough, the pain cut right through that. I do think it helped me start to relax though. Finally, after an hour, I told Jeff to get the nurse and bring on "the needle." I was hoping I had labored long enough and that the baby was in a good position so as not to bring on an unnecessary C-section. I will never forget getting the epidural. For me it was kind of funny because the narcotics were still working a bit. They told me to sit with my legs crossed to steady my back and then they raised the bed up for the anesthesiologist. As the bed was rising , I just couldn't NOT giggle. I felt like Buddha! Or some Buddhist god or goddess. So I sat like I was doing a meditation and kept telling Jeff that it felt like I was a floating Buddha hovering above the earth. Then the bed stopped and I let the guy give me an epidural.

Once it started working I tried to sleep. I told Jeff to sleep. He didn't until he thought I was actually asleep, worried that I might need him. I assured him it was fine with me and if he could get even a little rest that would be fantastic. At this point one of us needed to sleep, especially if the other couldn't (which I didn't). I passed in and out of weird dreams when I was half awake and, finally, it was 7:00 a.m. and the new L&D nurse came in.

Immediately, I was STARVING! Which made me feel nauseous. While pregnant, if I didn't eat in the morning, I'd get sick. I grabbed the nurse, who was delightful, and said, "I know you can't give me any food, but if I don't eat something, I'll throw up." She laughed (in a fun way, not mocking) and said, "Can't give you anything to eat!" and I responded, "Then grab that bowl! I need to throw up right now!" And I did.

Our doctor walked in soon after, around 8:00 a.m., with her infectious good nature and laughter. I told her I'd gotten sick last night as well and she said she also "threw up both of her babies." She immediately examined me and said, "You threw that baby right into position. You're ready to push!" Apparently, I had been in Transitional Labor. I had been thinking right before she came in that the baby probably wouldn't come until noon and how on earth would I ever survive that long without food! What great news that the baby was almost here!

I have to say, delivery was joyful and fun. I mean, I couldn't feel a thing! And our doctor is just funny and always in good spirits. GREAT energy! She told me to use my imagination to push and I also remembered Kathy had said, "Shoot for the light!" So I found a light on the ceiling and aimed! To the best of my imagination, at least.

Jeff was fascinated and watched the whole thing. All of a sudden the doctor cried out, "Elizabeth, give me your hand! Here, touch the head." I hadn't planned on doing that and it was amazing! I couldn't believe it! To be so close to meeting the baby! Not long after that, the doctor cried out again, "Elizabeth, reach down here with both your hands and pull your baby up!" I didn't even think about it, my hands reached out and I pulled the baby out and up onto my chest and announced that we had a boy! I looked at our baby boy in awe and then to Jeff. We both had tears in our eyes. I don't have words for that moment, but it is my favorite memory of the birth. I told my doctor the other day she had given me the greatest gift by letting me do that. I will never forget pulling him onto my chest. And I will never forget the look in Jeff's eyes. First touch. Instantly connected and in love. And then we watched Jeff cut the cord. Wyatt was so alert. He was looking all around, so curious! He had these big, beautiful, curious eyes.

At 8:45 a.m., we had a baby boy who weighed 6 lb 2oz.

I didn't get to spend very long with Wyatt right after the birth. He had a fever and I had a fever. They also thought he had amniotic fluid in his lungs. He was making a cute singing sound that, while cute, wasn't a great sign. I let Jeff know he could stand with the nurses while they were examining and weighing Wyatt, who was also a healthy crier, and sure enough, with Jeff standing close, the baby stopped crying but resumed that singing sound. The nurses were awesome though, and constantly kept reassuring us and keeping our spirits high. They then whisked Wyatt off to NICU for monitoring. By the time he got there, his fever was gone. His lungs were fine. But to be safe, they started him on antibiotics.

I tried to stay positive but I finally admitted to myself that it felt like I ran the marathon and WON, but no one would give me my winning "time" or the "medal." Then, I told myself, my baby is fine. They are just being cautious and how lucky is that? Some women leave here without a baby, and two friends of mine had miscarriages only a few months ago. I'm lucky. I have a baby that's healthy and we're being extra cautious with a little extra monitoring. So I "gave in" to the day and the reality that all will be ok even if it was not how I expected it to go. It was just weird because I felt as if I still didn't "know" he was mine—I only got a few minutes with him.

So Jeff and I spent the next day-and-a-half between the post-partum ward and NICU to be around Wyatt as much as possible and to breastfeed him every three hours. He was the healthiest baby in there so he was always the last to be checked by the doctor. Finally, he got to come to our room on Saturday at 3:00 p.m. We were so in awe when they wheeled him in! We kept saying, "We can't believe he's ours." It was such an amazing process of becoming an actual mom with an actual baby in my arms. Moving from awkward to empowered. Moving from being shy to knowing what I needed to do. Realizing he was ours. KNOWING he was ours. He was still alert and curious from birth to the NICU to our room. He loves to check everything out. He's very strong and peaceful for such a little guy.

I realized I had been waiting for this moment since I was about four or five years old and used to play with my dolls like I was a mother. I always loved babies and told my mom I wanted lots of them! I look at Wyatt and nothing else matters as much as our family; Jeff, Wyatt, and me. I look at him and realize this is why I'm here. I'm here to help bring him into the world. We are so lucky!

I look at my husband and I've never loved him more. I love him more in every way—as my love, my best friend, the father of our child and as my husband. He's sexier, stronger and just as perfect. He was born for this.

Wyatt to us means little adventurer, a guide. We hope to give him a life full of adventures or the opportunity for him to navigate through the adventures that will surely come his way. Already he seems like a little explorer—destined to the name that chose him. Because it did choose him.

And, finally, we've just been adjusting to our new, wonderful life. We can't remember life before Wyatt and it's been only two weeks. He is the most precious baby boy!! He's taken to breast-feeding like a champ and the way he eats, he'd better be an athlete! Goodness! And we've definitely had some adventures in "diaper changing" with a little boy. Wow.

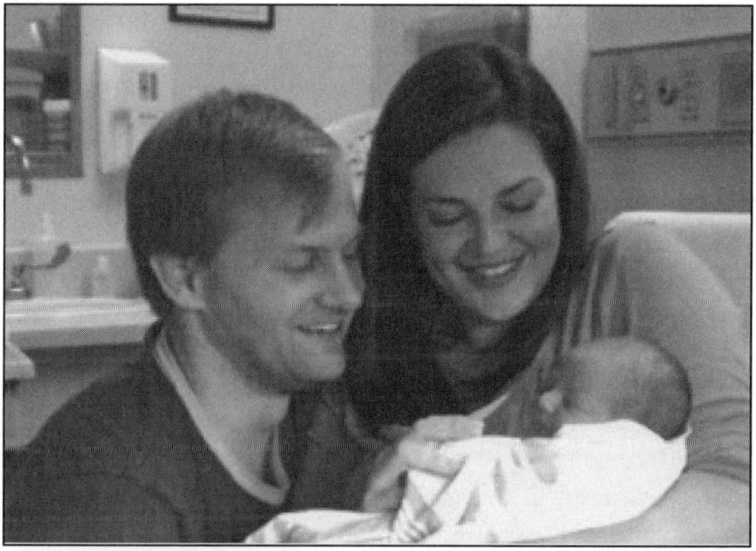

Elizabeth and Jeff welcome their first child, Wyatt.

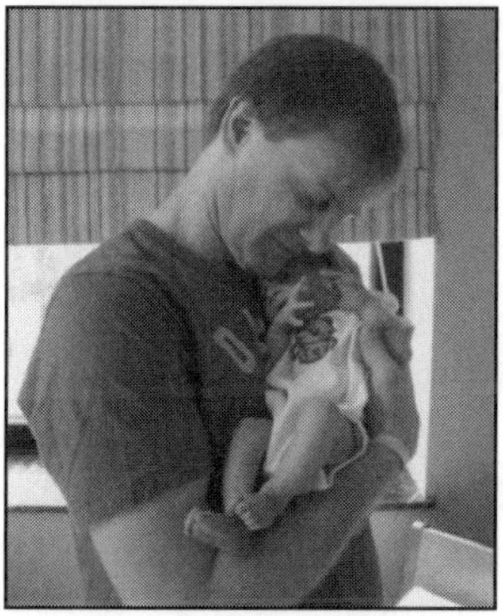

Jeff enjoys the fatherhood role early in the postpartum period.

Carson's Birth Story

Over the past two years, eight of my friends had precious little babies. Out of those, seven were delivered C-section. I had heard the C-section rate was high in the United States, around 30 percent, but this indicated more like 88 percent! Most of the stories were the same: after hours of labor, the fetal heart rate dropped, and the doctors had to do an emergency C-section. In the end, all of my friends were relieved to deliver healthy babies; however, almost all of them were disappointed with how their whole labor experience had unraveled. Not one mother left the hospital feeling that she had had control during those crucial hours.

When my turn finally came, I knew I didn't want to be part of that 88 percent. I understood that pregnancy and labor were unpredictable and that many things would not go my way. But I also knew there were steps I could take that would make me feel more in control and not at the mercy of the medicine and doctors. Hiring a doula and writing a birth plan were the two most valuable steps I took. During the first meeting with my doula, Kathy, we discussed my thoughts on how I envisioned the big day. Did I want any pain medication? What positions did I want to use? How did I feel about the tub or shower? Knowing that I did not want to lie in the hospital bed the entire time, these questions empowered me.

After completing my birth plan, the next step was to share it with my doctor. In my case, my OB was very respectful of my wishes and did everything she could to help me follow it. Upon entering the hospital on the day of my induction, my plan was immediately implemented. I wore my own clothes instead of a hospital gown, I walked the halls of the hospital for hours and used the birthing ball instead of lying in the bed, and I did squats and nipple stimulation to speed along the labor. At times when I hit a plateau and wasn't progressing, the doctors worked with me. The first doctor put me on Pitocin for a couple of hours to get me "jump started," but true to her word, when I started dilating, she took me off the medicine and let me jump into a warm shower! When I hit another plateau, the second doctor didn't even suggest Pitocin. Knowing my birth plan, she suggested that I change my position and lower my head below the cervix to relieve the pressure. The nurses adjusted the bed angle, I turned on all fours in a yoga position, and it worked! From then on, I was able to progress on my own with no drugs or IVs hooked up to me, just as I had hoped.

After thirteen hours of walking, squatting, twisting, and turning, my beautiful baby girl was finally born, and I truly felt blessed. So many things could have gone wrong that day, but they didn't. No fetal distress, no C-section. Who knows, maybe this would've all transpired the same way if I hadn't had a doula or a birth plan. Maybe it was just luck that things turned out my way. But I don't think so. Exhausted, I held my baby girl in my arms that day and sighed, "We did it."

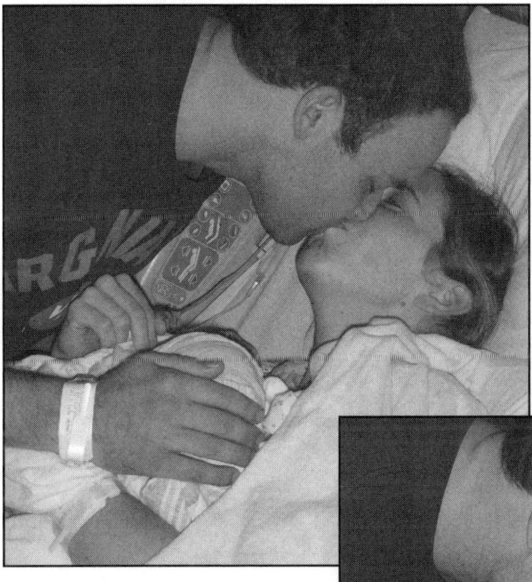

Jeremy kisses his wife, Allison, as they welcome their first child, Carson.

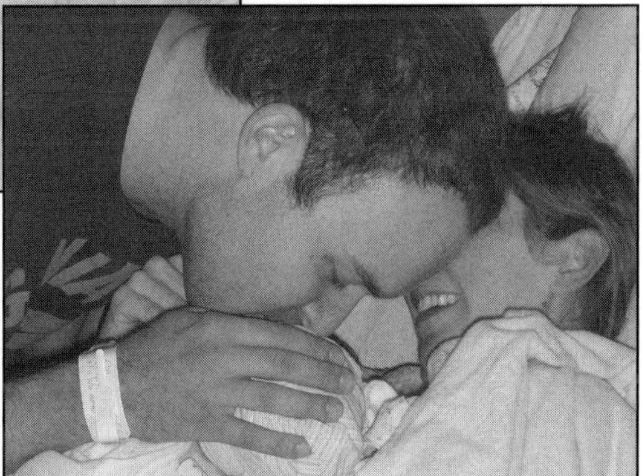

Jeremy is falling in love again as he gives his beautiful daughter her first kiss.

Maeve's Birth Story—Labor of Love

My husband and I were expecting our first daughter in October 2005. We were very excited. I always said that if I had a child I wanted to have an all natural birth, so we needed help in planning this out and coming up with a birth plan. I started doing some research as to different people who could help us and I came across a doula. I didn't even know what a doula was, or what they did, but I read more and thought this is perfect for us. A doula is there to help you in the writing of the birth plan and to guide things along when in the hospital. After our experience, I am a firm believer that a doula and a birth plan are essential to a smooth birthing experience.

We interviewed half a dozen doulas and when we met Kathy we knew in our hearts she was the doula for us. Not only did she have years of experience but she was also a pediatric nurse practitioner and had a strong sense of self. She helped us have everything we ever wanted in a birth. We met a few months into my pregnancy and went over all my wishes of how I wanted my labor and birth to go. I also took a Lamaze class that she taught.

Having a doula involved in my birth plan made me feel confident and well prepared. We had our plan and a back-up plan, in case my original plan didn't follow through. I learned I was the first patient in the hospital to have a mirror in the operating room when I had my C-section performed, as I didn't want to miss out on the birth of my daughter. Kathy made this happen for me and was my voice in my time of need. My husband also got to experience the birth while our doula took care of the details, which took so much pressure off both of us.

We delivered a beautiful baby girl. After the birth, Kathy provided postpartum services to our family that were as significant as being our doula during my pregnancy. I had some medical complications and didn't have family nearby. Kathy helped me immensely in the transition of coming home and my new role as a mother in the early days after my daughter's birth and the months afterward. She helped me breastfeed, provided me with great rest and support. Our professional relationship turned into an everlasting friendship which we will always hold dearly in our hearts. Kathy will always be part of our family.

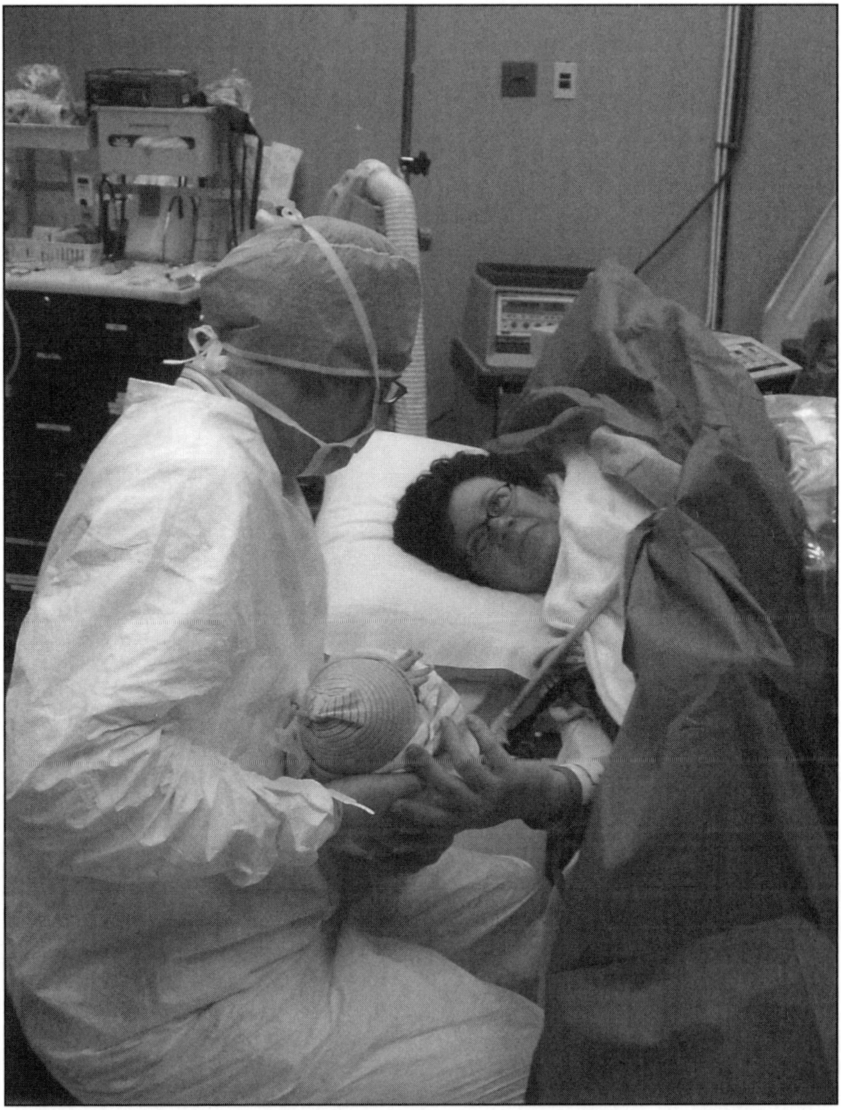

Jennifer and Ger share an excited glance at each other while welcoming their daughter, Maeve.

Kaysen, Henley and Louisa's Birth Stories

I've had three deliveries, each of them quite different. While my birth plans were similar for all three, each experience impacted the next birth plan. For my first delivery, I was adamantly against being induced or having any unnecessary medical interventions. I hoped to be able to have a drug-free birth, so my husband and I hired a doula and signed up for a Lamaze class. My labor started ten days before my due date, and I spent about thirty hours enjoying the early stages before heading to the hospital. It was great—my husband and I went shopping for a new camera, we went out to eat, we walked around the outdoor mall, I fed the horses, and we watched a movie, and all the while, I was stopping every few minutes to breathe through my contractions. Our doula had prepared us well for what to expect, and we were perfectly content to stay away from the hospital as long as possible.

When I couldn't stand the pain anymore, we drove the forty-five minutes to the hospital. To my surprise, I was only a "dimple" dilated! They were about to send me home when my water broke and the fun really began.

I labored a couple of hours in the shower, but the back pain was overwhelming and I was exhausted from not having slept the past two nights. I asked for the epidural and was shocked to find out that I had to receive a whole bag of fluids before they could administer it, which took about forty-five minutes. Big lesson learned: in my next birth, I made sure I got hooked up to the fluids as soon as possible, just in case!

I was six or seven centimeters dilated when I finally got some relief, and it was heaven. I had no idea that I could sleep through labor, which was exactly what I did for the next few hours. The thing that really scared me was the pushing—I didn't know how long it would take or how painful it would be, particularly since my baby was "sunny-side-up" (positioned to deliver face-up), and very high up in the birth canal. I never felt the urge to push, so I was able to wait comfortably until the doctor was ready. Once I started, it took only about twenty minutes to bring my first daughter into the world. I held her for a few minutes, but she was grunting, so they took her away to the nursery where they checked and bathed her. I didn't see her for four hours! Because of the epidural, I had to wait awhile before I could get out of bed, so I certainly couldn't tromp down to the nursery to find her. Another lesson learned!

Nineteen months later, I found myself in labor with my second child. Again, everything started ten days before my due date. Without any contractions or any type of warning, I lost my mucus plug. We had hired the same doula that we used with our first child, who by that point had become a close friend. She had told us that, in general, delivery of the second child occurs forty-eight hours after losing the mucus plug. She was exactly right! For two days, I had contractions (back labor, of course) off and on. Most of this time was spent at home on my hands and knees, trying to get the baby to turn into the head-down position.

At about 4 p.m. on the second day, my contractions suddenly got intense. While waiting for my in-laws to come, I got into the tub with my daughter and enjoyed some relief in the warm water. On the way to the hospital, I drank two ounces of champagne from a paper cup because we had been told that a little champagne would relax me. (I didn't drink at all during my pregnancy, but I was willing to try a little for delivery.) It worked like a charm!

By the time I got to the hospital around 7 p.m., my contractions had reduced in intensity. I thought maybe they would send me home, but it turns out that I was seven centimeters dilated and 80 percent effaced! I had updated my birth plan to indicate that I wanted to labor in the tub and that I did not want to have to get back into bed for monitoring for at least an hour and a half. I had received my OB's blessing on this wish, as well. Everything went perfectly—I was in the tub for an hour until I started to feel pressure, and then I got out and delivered my second daughter in two pushes. Unbelievably, it didn't even hurt to push her out! I had also included in my birth plan that I did not want my baby taken away to the nursery to be weighed and bathed, so I got to breastfeed her and keep her with me for hours after her birth. I showered and walked myself to the room—what a treat it was to be able to feel and use my legs so soon after delivery.

After the incredible experience I had giving birth to my second daughter, I thought my third would be a breeze. My birth plan was very similar to my second, with the added request that my child not be bathed until the next day to allow me even more time to bond. While I was able to keep my third daughter (yes, three girls!) with me until the next day, the rest of the delivery didn't quite go as expected.

Again, I started having contractions off and on, a couple days in advance, and it took me a long time to get into active labor. I thought things would move pretty fast, so I stayed close to the hospital, going to Starbucks and walking around a nearby mall. I had a doctor's appointment scheduled for mid-afternoon, and when I went in, I was five centimeters dilated. I wanted to continue to labor on my own, but the nurse said my blood pressure was high and I was sent immediately to the hospital.

At the hospital, my blood pressure was normal, but the baby's heart rate was elevated, so I stayed hooked to the monitor for several hours. I was able to labor on the ball and in a rocking chair, but I couldn't walk around or get in the shower, and the room I was in had no tub. The reason the baby's heart rate was elevated was because the heat system was broken and it was at least ninety degrees in the labor and delivery room! Several workmen came in and finally fixed the heat, at which point the baby's heart rate was normal, and they released me from the monitor.

As with my previous birth plans, I had indicated that I did not want my water broken, but my doctor kept pressuring me to rupture the bag of water. I finally gave in around 5:00 p.m. because she said she would not stick around all night to deliver me. After my water was broken, I was able to walk around a little, so I did one loop of the labor-delivery ward. Huffing and puffing through contractions, I put on quite a show for the people who were looking at the new babies in the nursery. When I got back to the room, the pressure was very intense and I was ready to push. The nurse checked me and I was only nine centimeters, so I was instructed to "blow little candles" to prevent pushing. It was intolerable, and I cried and screamed that I couldn't do it. My doctor had taken a dinner break and was unavailable, and I wasn't going to be allowed to push until she returned. Fortunately, after what seemed like forever but was probably only five minutes, she returned and allowed me to push. As with my second, it took only one or two pushes to get her out, but this time it was quite painful!

In general, I would say that the delivery was a good one—I did not need an epidural or any other serious medical intervention—but it was a lot less "natural" than my second delivery in that I was not able to do things on my own terms. I think this

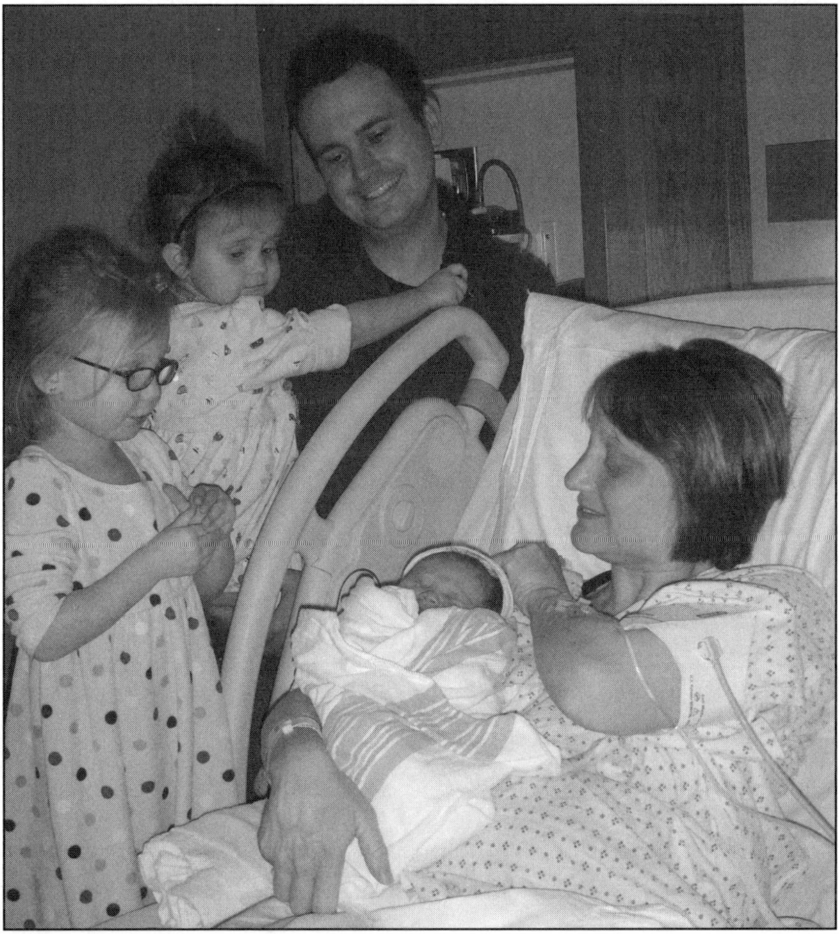

Daddy Wray is now surrounded by all females, with baby #3 another girl, Louisa. Kaysen and Henley are thrilled with their new sister.

had a significant impact on my perception of the pain. If I were to have a fourth child, which at this point I don't think I will, I would strongly consider having it in a non-hospital setting so that I could avoid some of the issues I had with my third delivery.

My birth plan played a significant role in all three of my deliveries. It was a very effective tool for communicating my desires with my doula, the nurses, and my doctor. I experienced what I would consider the "perfect" hospital delivery with my second, and I attribute this to two things: a great doula and a great birth plan. My first and third deliveries did not go exactly as I had planned, but I do believe having a good birth plan made them go as well as possible. I was particularly happy to be able to bond with my newborn daughters for a lot longer than normal for a hospital delivery and, in all three situations, I really enjoyed the whole childbirth experience.

Lula's Birth Story

My pregnancy with my daughter Lula was full of anxiety, worry, and cautious hope. Our son, Theo, had died a year-and-a-half earlier of a rare and aggressive brain tumor at nine months old. Having since become very active in support groups for families whose children and babies have died, and having heard so many other heartbreaking stories, it seems I know nearly every way a baby can die. And once you have been a statistic, statistics don't go very far in making you feel better about the laws of probability. Still, I felt that if we did not have another child, my husband and I would regret it in later years. I wanted a baby.

When I gave birth to my son, my wish was for a completely natural childbirth with no interventions. I labored for twenty-four hours naturally until finally I agreed to have first, Pitocin, in an attempt to coax my cervix into opening those last few centimeters, and then, when that didn't work (and after pain much worse than I had experienced without the Pitocin), I had an epidural in an attempt to avoid a C-section. The labor was thirty-six hours total. Luckily, I did get to give birth vaginally and when my doctor came in and announced that I was finally ten centimeters dilated, we dialed down the epidural meds and I was able to have some control over pushing. It felt great to finally be able to have some control over my body and the birthing process. When Theo's head and shoulders came out, my doctor told me to reach down and pull my baby out. I did and it was one of the best feelings I have ever had. He was beautiful.

I was lucky to have had two wonderful doulas who took shifts with me. Every pregnant and laboring woman should have a doula! One stayed with us all night long from the time of our arrival at the hospital around 8:30 p.m., and the other came in around 10:00 a.m. and stayed with us until our son was born the following day at two minutes past midnight.

During those long, painful hours, my husband's mother died of a stroke. He was exhausted, shocked and grief stricken in the midst of the arrival of our son. And, of course, we had no way of knowing then that our sweet baby boy, our first born child, would also die before his first birthday of a terribly aggressive brain tumor.

I knew when I became pregnant with Lula, two years later, that I would need people around me who could support me unconditionally, who had also known Theo, who knew all we had been through, and who would understand my particular anxieties and fears, as well as my wishes for my daughter's birth. Kathy Stewart in her capacity of nurse practitioner was Theo's primary healthcare practitioner until the tragedy of brain cancer struck our family. She saw him on his first visit to the pediatrician and for the next three months until he was diagnosed with the tumor. She came to visit him when he was in the PICU and was a source of compassionate support throughout his illness. For the birth of our daughter, I knew there was no one else I would have wanted to be there with us except Kathy.

For the birth of my daughter, I would love to have had a home birth in the water, but my fears of losing another baby to an unforeseen turn of events, no matter how unlikely, made it impossible for me to choose that course. In addition, I had decided several weeks before her due date to have an epidural simply because I wanted a peaceful and easeful transition for her into this world. After the long and painful labor I experienced with Theo's birth, I wanted this birth to be different, less stressful and less frightening. I also greatly wanted my husband to have a peaceful experience during the birth of our second child. I knew that my pregnancy was just as scary for him as it was for me. We were both terrified that something awful would happen. I had only my previous experiences with which to compare, and I was convinced that labor with my second child would be just as long as it had been for my first baby. I knew how hard it was for my husband to see me in such pain for such a prolonged time and under such stressful circumstances. The memory was a difficult one for him. I also wanted my longtime ob-gyn to attend this birth, as she had Theo's. Therefore, for all those reasons, I had to have a hospital birth. But I still wanted as few interventions as possible while maintaining safety for my baby and trying to ensure, as far as possible, a safe delivery.

I expressed all my concerns, fears and wishes to Kathy, who understood everything perfectly. When I told her I was certain that this birth would be just as long and painful as Theo's had been nearly three years earlier, she told me that second babies usually come in about half the time of first babies (and eighteen hours did sound much better than thirty-six).

Then Kathy told me, "But we're just putting it out to the universe that this birth will take only eight hours." She nodded knowingly.

I raised my eyebrows, laughed and said, "Ok, let's put it out there." I had my doubts, but something in me wanted to believe that if she said it, it just might come true. She made it easy to think that the universe just might listen. She also made it very easy for me to feel good about my decisions and my choices and to trust in my own intuition.

Lula's due date was May 1. Theo had been born a week before his due date. Again, having nothing else to compare it to, I thought, and hoped, that Lula might also come a little early. When there were no signs of her impending arrival the week before, I began doing all the old wives' tales tricks that supposedly help to "kick-start" labor. Nothing happened. I went to an acupuncturist who specializes in a holistic approach to pregnancy. The session was very relaxing. I felt calm and peaceful. Later that night, I felt some movement, some shifting around, some discomfort, and had some slight, pinkish discharge, but no real labor yet. We went again for a second treatment the following morning, the day before the due date, hoping the second treatment would serve to set my labor in motion. I felt as if I were floating on the table. It was a wonderful, peaceful feeling.

In addition to the second acupuncture treatment, we had an appointment to see our doctor late that afternoon. I had purposefully scheduled the appointment at the end of the day on April 30, the day before our due date. My doctor and I had discussed ways of attempting to induce labor without the use of Pitocin. Having had a terrible, painful experience with Pitocin before, it was high on my list of things to try my best to avoid, second only to a C-section. She knew my fears of going overdue, as well as my wishes to avoid interventions as far as possible. She suggested placing prostaglandin gel inside my cervix which, we discovered at the appointment, was dilated a little less than a centimeter. Usually, the insertion of prostaglandin gel can start natural labor within six to twelve hours. We did this in a labor and delivery room, just in case we needed to stay. After the insertion of the gel, I had to lie completely still for an hour to see if it worked. She placed the gel and left with instructions to call in two hours or so if it worked, or if it didn't. I didn't know what we were going to do if it didn't work. I imagined we might go home and wait another day. I was worried and anxious about going past the due date, though, and wanted to see my baby here safe and sound.

After about thirty minutes, I began to feel the first twinges of cramps, which developed very quickly into full-blown contractions. An hour after the gel was placed I was in serious labor! My husband and I walked the circuit around Labor & Delivery, passing by the nurses' station and other rooms, over and over, stopping to grab hold of the bars along the walls and breathe through contractions every fifteen minutes or so. At around 9:00 p.m., we called Kathy, who came to the hospital right away. We went on like that for a while, walking, stopping for contractions, breathing, sitting on the birthing ball, trying various positions of sitting, standing, moving, breathing. With each full-on contraction, I continued to be amazed at how much it hurt. I had forgotten how painful it really was, even though I told myself I would never forget how much that hurt!

After being checked around 9:30 p.m. at about three centimeters, I decided to go ahead and get the epidural. I was sure it was going to be a long night. I thought it would be nice to be able to rest, relax, maybe get some sleep and have a baby with the sunrise. The anesthesiologist arrived at about quarter to ten and I was lying comfortably in the bed by 10:45 or so, ready to sleep for a bit, figuring that the baby would come around early morning.

My husband went home to let the dog out, feed the cats and get a few things for the night and the hospital stay. I told Kathy, as she sat in the rocking chair next to the bed, that she should go home and get some sleep, too, since there was no sense in her staying here all night for no reason. She should just come back early and be here for the birth in the morning.

She shook her head and said, "Oh, no, girl! That baby's gonna be here in a few hours." I laughed, raised my eyebrows, shook my head and replied, "Ok, but I doubt it. I wish you would get some sleep." But I didn't argue. I would rather have had her there anyway.

She told me to try to rest while I could, and I decided to follow her advice. Some quiet minutes later, I was about to drop off to sleep when I felt a huge POP! and an enormous, wet, warm gush between my legs. I gasped and woke completely out of my sleepy, relaxed state.

"Oh my God! I think my water just broke!"

When my water broke before the birth of our son, I had experienced a steady, but relatively small, trickle of amniotic fluid down my leg. His head was sufficiently covering the cervical opening so that the water came out only a bit at a time. This powerful, immediate surge of water was different and completely unexpected.

Kathy got the nurse, who did a check, looked up at me, and said, "You are about nine centimeters dilated."

WHAT?! I could not believe it! Kathy started laughing and I was frantically dialing the phone to get my husband who wasn't answering. As soon as I said, "He must be on his way," he walked in the door. He was just as surprised to hear the news. The nurse left to call our doctor and soon there was a hustle and bustle of activity in the room. The setting up of the instruments, the bringing in of the equipment, the tearing open of sterile packages of various things and implements. As I watched all of this going on around me, I began to feel a deep pressure that seemed to be saying "Push, Push" and I told Kathy about it. She and the nurses kept asking me how I felt, told me not to push yet, asked whether I felt like I needed to push, kept telling me "It's almost time!" As each second passed, I kept feeling more and more the urge to push.

Our doctor came quickly into the room, pulling on her gloves, slid onto her stool, checked inside, looked up, smiled, and said, "Ten centimeters!" I began to push.

At 1:40 a.m. on May 1, after just a little over seven hours of labor, Lula Frances was born! I watched in the mirror as her head emerged. Her eyes were wide open. The nurses said she was looking around at everything in the room, and then, almost immediately after her head was born, her right shoulder, arm and hand slung out in a wide arc. It looked exactly like she'd thrown her arm out in a cheerful wave, as if to say, "Hello, world! Here I am!"

Lula is now two years old. She has had that open, exuberant, high-spirited attitude since the very first moment of her arrival. The universe heard. We were granted not only a less than eight-hour labor, but a beautiful, healthy, perfect baby girl who has brought immeasurable joy to our hearts.

In no way does Lula take the place of our son, and her birth is not the "happy ending" that I think some people imagined it would be, or maybe should be. One child does not substitute for another. It is a strange thing to be able to hold such heartache and elation at the same time in the space of one heart. Joy next to pain, happiness alongside grief. When I held Lula in my arms for the first time, I knew immediately the magic trick that a parent has of being able to completely and totally, and with the whole heart, love more than one child at once. It is an amazing feat. We appear to be a family of three, but will always be a family of four. We have not one child, but two. Lula will know about her brother as she grows—she already recognizes his pictures and calls him "Bruver." And I know, without a doubt, that he knows her and that he is proud to have such a wonderful little sister to watch over.

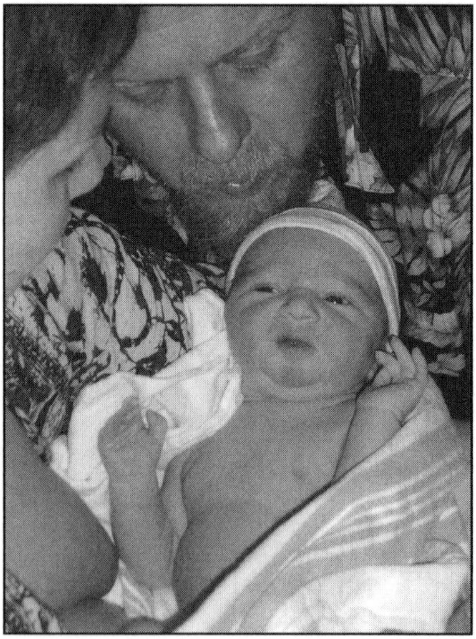

Lula is alert and looking around as parents Karla and Jamie gaze at their beautiful daughter.

Asher's Birth Story

When I sat down to write our birth plan, I had visions of everything going according to the "plan." Needless to say, it did not happen that way! Even though the birth of our son, Asher, did not go as planned, it was still one of the most beautiful moments of our lives. Second only to our doula, the birth plan was the most valuable tool in helping make our birthing experience run smoothly. The writing of the plan alone caused us to research our options and allowed us to discuss with our doctor the pros and cons of those options. We went into the birth experience being educated, which I think goes a long way to making one feel more comfortable when the day arrives. We were able to formulate a birth plan that we felt best suited our wants and needs. On the big day, the birth plan allowed the hospital staff to be aware of what our plan was for the birthing process and helped them better care for us. It assured us that everyone involved would be on the same page and there was no need to make hasty decisions. It also allowed the staff to know that we knew what options were available to us and that any deviations from the plan would come from us. I think the most valuable aspect of using a birth plan is the dialog it creates between you and your doctor or midwife prior to the birth.

The only thing I would have changed about my birth plan is that I would make sure my doctor and I were on the same page about how long after my due date the practice would allow me to go. The OB practice said they do not let women go past forty-one weeks. I had written in my birth plan that I did not want to discuss induction until I was at forty-two weeks. When the doctor saw that in the birth plan she would not sign it until I made the change. I made the change thinking that there was no way I would go that long. At forty-one weeks we still had no baby and I was scheduled for an induction. It was hard to negotiate with the doctor at this point; all negotiations should be done well in advance of the due date. Looking back on it, I really believe that my labor was so hard and long (I think I pushed for over two hours) because my little guy was not ready to come into the world yet.

Overall, the birth plan really helped my husband and me discuss what it was that we wanted from our birthing experience. It helped us communicate those wants to our doctor. And it ultimately gave me peace during labor that we were all working together from the same blueprint.

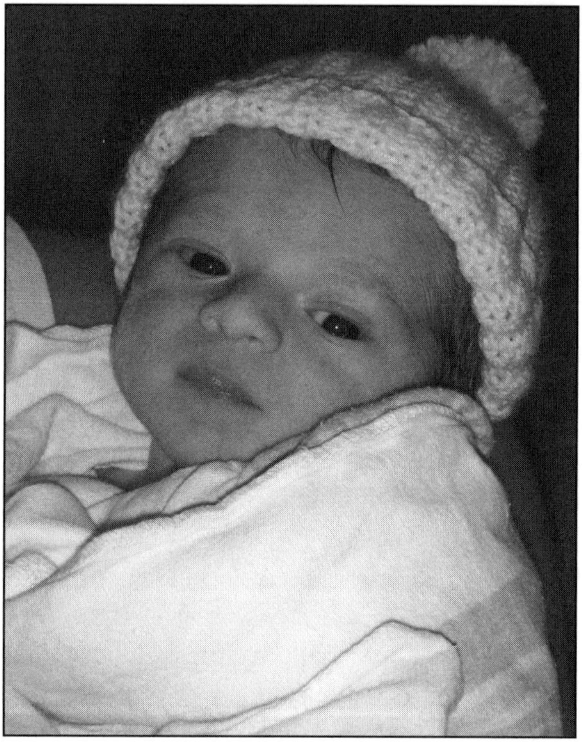

Just a few minutes old, Asher has captured the hearts of his parents, Beth and Josh.

Evan's Birth Story

I had a 39-week appointment on October 1 at 11:45 a.m. Jeff went with me and I had asked our midwife to go ahead and check my cervix. The last time my cervix had been checked prior to this appointment was at 37 weeks. At that 37-week appointment I had been 1+ cm dilated and 50 percent effaced. Since then I had been having intense Braxton Hicks and cramping, so I was hoping that meant I was progressing.

The Braxton Hicks and cramping subsided a day or two before the 39-week appointment. Our midwife proceeded to check me and had a hard time locating my cervix. She warned me that if I wasn't cramping then, I would be after the exam. We even half-joked about the exam kick-starting labor through all the poking and prodding! Once she was able to locate my cervix, she said she wished she had more encouraging news. I was still a little over 1 cm, maybe 2 cm dilated and 60 percent effaced. Jeff and I were a little disappointed but knew that our little one would be here when he was ready. We wouldn't be pregnant forever!

After the appointment, we decided to go to lunch together before heading back to work. At lunch, I started cramping, and toward the end of lunch, the cramping got a little stronger. I just thought it was from the exam and nothing more.

I returned to work at 1:30 p.m., and the cramps became more intense—starting in the back and continuing to the front—and they seemed to be coming at regular intervals. I could feel my uterus tightening. I just couldn't believe that I could be having actual contractions or that I was in labor, but I started to time them, and they were 8 to 10 minutes apart. I called our midwife and left her a message.

I stayed at work for an hour timing the contractions, still not wanting to believe that I was actually in labor. I finally decided that it was time to leave work. I called our midwife on her cell phone as I drove home. She asked if I wanted to come in to be checked but she said that she wasn't too hopeful that I would be more dilated than I was this morning. We decided that I would go home since I was already almost there and call her again when my contractions were 4 to 5 minutes apart.

When I got home at 3:30, my contractions still continued at 8 to 10 minutes apart. Jeff got home with our daughter around 4:45 p.m. and my mother-in-law took care of her while I stayed in our room.

At around 5:00 o'clock, I called our midwife to let her know that my contractions were pretty intense and were coming regularly at 4 to 5 minutes. She was amazed at my progress and said she guessed she may have actually started something up during my appointment! We agreed to meet at the hospital at Labor and Delivery at 6:30 p.m. She said she would call ahead to let them know that I was coming.

At around 5:45 p.m., my contractions seemed to be coming more quickly, but I wasn't timing them at this point. I was putting all my focus on laboring. My husband got everything in the car. I started getting anxious to leave for the hospital. I wanted to let our daughter know I was leaving and that I loved her. I knew I had only a brief break between contractions to get with her. I didn't want her to see me during a contraction. At 6:10 p.m., I told her we were leaving, and we headed out the door.

When we arrived at the hospital at 6:30, I was completely unaware that my contractions were coming 2 to 3 minutes apart. I knew they were coming pretty fast but I wasn't in any mind to track them and my husband was concentrating on driving without hitting a lot of bumps on the way. Jeff pulled up to the front entrance and there just happened to be a volunteer with a wheelchair heading back into the hospital. I knew I wouldn't be able to walk to Labor and Delivery, so I asked the volunteer to assist me and he wheeled me up to L & D while my husband parked the car.

The nurses proceeded to get me set up. I answered questions and signed what I could between contractions. They needed to get me into bed to monitor the baby and my contractions for 15 minutes. The bed was very uncomfortable and I knew this would make labor a little more difficult. I did finally get into bed so they could put me on a monitor. Once I was on the monitor, the midwife said my contractions were 2 to 3 minutes apart and she wanted to know when they started at that interval. I told her about 5:45 p.m. She wanted to check me and said the nursing staff may have to wait on the other things they needed to do. She checked my cervix and I was 8½ to 9 cm and 80 percent effaced. I started contracting and she asked how I felt, other than pain. I told her I had lots of pressure in my pelvic area and felt like I needed to go to the bathroom, and had felt that way since leaving the house. She then told the nursing staff that we were going to be delivering the baby within the next 30 minutes. They started getting ready for the birth.

She asked me if I wanted to push, and I said sure. She said, "If it feels good, let's keep pushing, if not, stop." With my next contraction, I started pushing and she checked me again and coached me along the way. Pushing felt very good! So I continued to push during each contraction.

Forty-five minutes after arriving at the hospital, Evan was born, at 7:31 p.m. He was 7 lb and 20¼ inches long. I had amazing birth experiences with both my children! I feel extremely blessed beyond compare with my children and the truly remarkable labor and delivery of each.

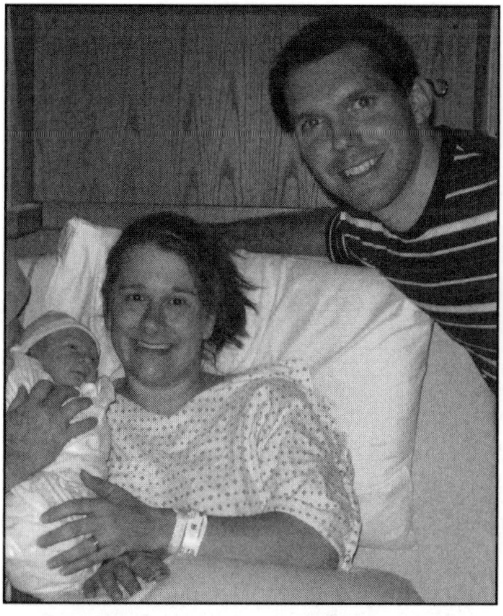

Jeff and Tammy are proud parents to baby boy, Evan.

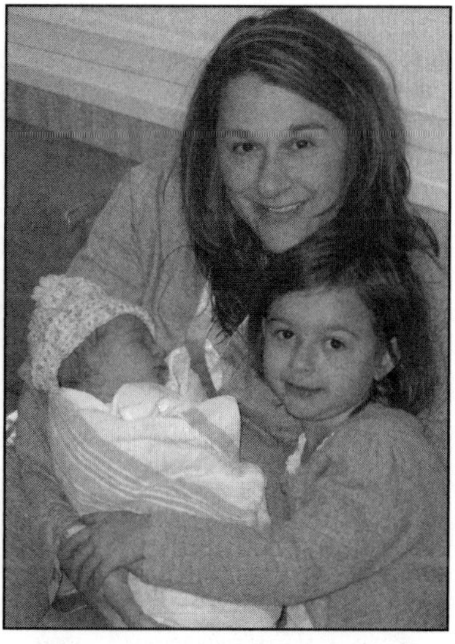

Big sister is excited about the arrival of her brother.

James' Birth Story

My due date was August 2, so I was ready, but not overly anxious when I woke around 5:00 a.m. on that Tuesday with contractions coming about ten minutes apart. I waited an hour before I woke my husband and we decided to just continue our day like we normally would in case this was a false alarm. My daughter woke up soon after and we all got ready for our day, putting the family on "red alert."

By 8:00 a.m. my contractions were stronger and about five minutes apart. Luckily, we were already on our way to take our daughter to the sitter's, and by the time we dropped her off, I called my midwife to let her know we were on the way to the hospital. Contractions were strong but not unbearable; however, they were coming closer together, so I wanted to get to my midwife as soon as possible. I was so excited, but still unwilling to believe I was truly in labor!

When I got to the hospital, my entire family was already there waiting for me in the visitor's room. No surprise there, we do everything together! We were all laughing and joking around while I filled out paperwork. The women behind the desk must have thought I was in the early stages and were unsure as to whether I was actually going to be admitted or sent home.

By 9:00 a.m., I was in the room being monitored by the nurses and my midwife was on her way. She got there soon after and checked me and I was pleasantly surprised to find out I was 8 cm, 100 percent effaced and the baby was at 0 station! Yea! He was on his way! I was still feeling really good between contractions although they were getting stronger and longer. I moved around a lot, and my husband applied counter pressure to my back during contractions. He was so supportive and really remembered everything we learned in our conscious birthing class! My mother was there, as well, a little nervous, but very supportive. The whole concept of a natural childbirth was a little scary to her.

After spending a few minutes on the birth ball, I got into the tub and that felt great. But soon after, I started feeling the pressure in my bottom getting more intense. The midwife checked me and I was fully dilated! I got out of the tub and immediately got on hands and knees and started pushing. That was really intense and, as I told my midwife, the phrase "urge to push" is the biggest understatement ever. It is so much more than an "urge"! It's a necessity.

When my arms were tired of holding up my body, I moved to a side-lying position and my son was crowning before long. The "ring of fire" phase was really tough because we were doing small pushes to ease him out slowly in the hopes of minimizing tearing since I had scar tissue from an episiotomy during my first birth. Before I knew it, his head was out. I saw that sweet face and the rest of him followed quickly. It was amazing and beautiful, and the best, hardest thing I have ever done.

James Roy was born at 12:01 p.m., after just three hours of hospital laboring! A big, healthy boy at 8 lb 12 oz and 20½ inches long.

Thank you so much for the education and help concerning childbirth. It was invaluable and key in my having a natural experience.

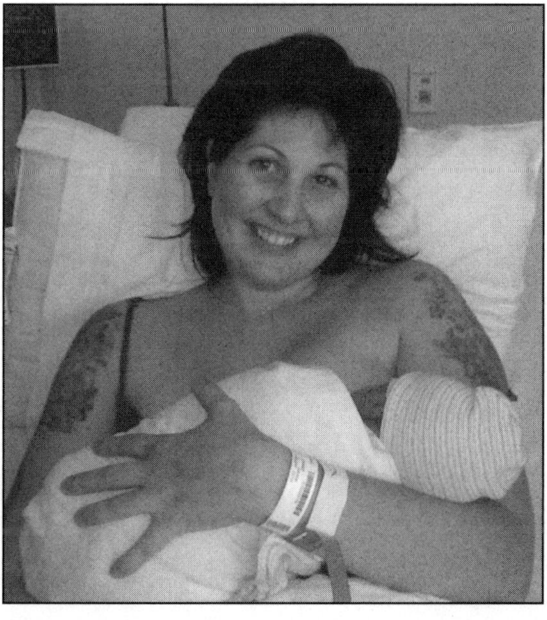

Chastity and her husband, Russell, welcomed their son, James Roy.

Reagan's Birth Story

Reagan was born 3 weeks early on March 31. We knew he was going to come early because at my 36-week appointment I was already 3 cm dilated and 80 percent effaced. My doctor asked me to rest so I could make it to 37 weeks (full term). Instead of resting, this news caused me to go into a crazy nesting tailspin! Despite this, we managed to make it to 37 weeks and 3 hours.

It was 3:00 a.m. on March 30 when I woke up to my water breaking. The good news was that we would have our little baby boy within 24 hours (knowing how concerned doctors are about infection after the water breaks). The bad news was that I wasn't in labor. I was having mild contractions every 10–15 minutes. I really wanted to avoid any interventions, so when we got to the hospital my husband (and amazing Lamaze coach) and I immediately started walking the floors in hopes of inducing labor.

At 8:00 a.m. my doctor arrived to examine me. Her first question was, "Do you feel as comfortable as you look?" I tried to convince her (and myself) that my contractions had gotten stronger, but my relaxed face and the monitors told otherwise. Despite our best efforts, we hadn't managed to start any "real" contractions and I was still around 3 cm dilated. They ended up starting the Pitocin drip at 10:00 a.m. Thankfully, with only a small dose, I started having strong contractions every 1–2 minutes.

My doctor checked me at around 12:30 p.m. I was 5 cm dilated and very relieved to be making progress. She told us that we would likely have the baby by 5:00 o'clock if I progressed at the typical 1 cm per hour. With this news, our nurses decided to take a lunch break…and so did my husband. He ordered a sandwich and asked my mother to take over for him for a quick break. Before the sandwich arrived, however, my labor began to escalate.

By 1:30 p.m. I started feeling the urge to push and had some of the signs of transition, like shaking and more intense contractions. My husband asked a nurse to come check me and I was at 7 cm. I knew things must be moving quickly when she started preparing the delivery table. By the time my nurse returned at

2:00 p.m., I was at 9 cm and they were calling the doctor. My body had started to push involuntarily and I couldn't stop it despite my best attempts at breathing the urge away.

As soon as the doctor arrived I started to actively push. By the second contraction, I understood what was meant by the "ring of fire" as his head came out. And, with the next contraction, our little boy arrived! Needless to say, my husband never got his sandwich!

What an amazing experience! It continues to awe me as I look at my sweet little boy!

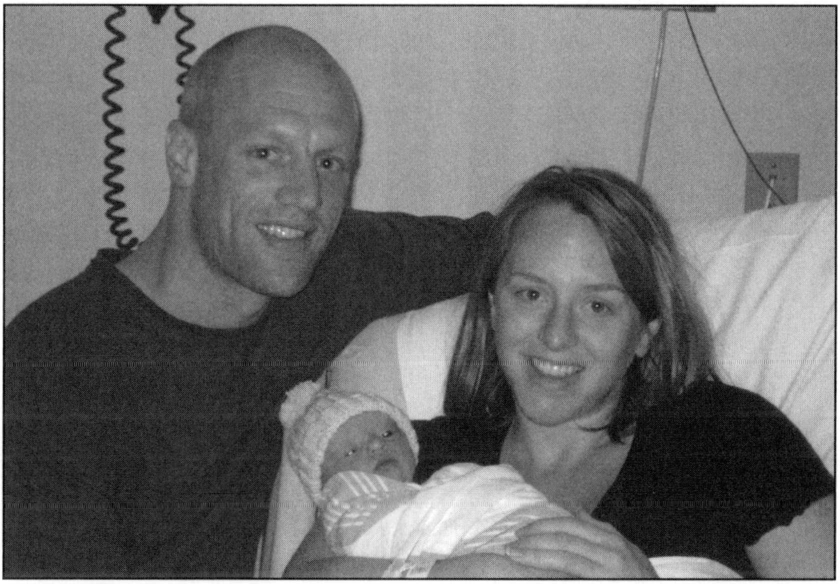

Chrissy and Paul are proud parents of their first son, Reagan.

Liberty "Libby" Grace's Birth Story

On April 30, 2010, at 7 a.m., two weeks before my due date, I woke up with mild contractions which wasn't unusual since I'd been having Braxton Hicks contractions for weeks. As I had gotten in the habit of doing, I started watching the clock and realized my contractions were coming pretty consistently every ten minutes. Since this was not my first pregnancy, I was particularly sensitive to having a "false alarm" since that would mean calling in the grandparents to watch our two-year-old son. Also, my water broke three weeks early with my first pregnancy, so I wasn't quite sure what "going into labor" felt like.

At 9 a.m. my son and I stopped by the local coffee shop on our way to the park for a neighborhood play-date. Midway through I started having difficulty holding a conversation and realized my contractions were close to six minutes apart. I decided to head into the doctor's office for an exam. My husband came home from work at noon to watch our son and, still determined not to have a false alarm, I drove myself over to the doctor's office, stopping on the way to fill up my car with gas. While I was filling up, a woman said, "You're about to have that baby any minute!" She didn't know how right she was.

When I arrived at the office, my nurse practitioner hooked me up to a monitor and confirmed that my contractions were five minutes apart, but when she examined me I had not made any progress since my last visit several days earlier. I was still about 2 centimeters dilated and 80 percent effaced. She explained that while I was having contractions, they weren't productive. She recommended I head home and remain active, hopefully encouraging more productive contractions. The baby's heart rate was a little too steady though, which can be a sign of fetal distress, so she asked me to stay for another hour to observe. Baby responded well to the sugary drink they gave me, but I became noticeably more uncomfortable and flushed. My nurse practitioner decided to examine me before I left and it's a good thing she did because I had progressed to 4 centimeters in less than an hour and was 90 percent effaced. This was no false alarm!

I was admitted to labor and delivery at 2 p.m. and my contractions were about four minutes apart. They were getting more intense, but I was still able to move around and visit with a friend while I waited for my husband (and labor coach) to arrive. He was there for about a half hour before I developed symptoms of transition—intense back pressure, shaking, and contractions 1-2 minutes apart. My doctor examined me at 4 p.m. and I was 7 centimeters and 100 percent effaced. Because of the intensity of my contractions, she anticipated that I would progress quickly. Within the hour, I started feeling the intense urge to push, but the nurses urged me to use the "blow out the candle" breathing technique to resist the urge because I wasn't quite 10 cm and pushing could cause swelling. At about 5 p.m., the nurse confirmed I had made it to 10 centimeters and called the doctor.

As soon as the doctor arrived, she gave me the go ahead to begin pushing. At this point, I started having second thoughts about declining the epidural as I imagined pushing out a big baby. Several days earlier, at my doctor visit, they estimated that I would have a 9-pound baby which was huge compared to my 5-pound 15-ounce first child. After my second push, I was so relieved to hear the doctor say, "You're almost there." That gave me the motivation I needed to push through the "ring of fire" and, at 5:20 p.m., meet our 6-pound, 11-ounce daughter, Liberty Grace. What a miracle and joy it has been to welcome little Libby into our family!

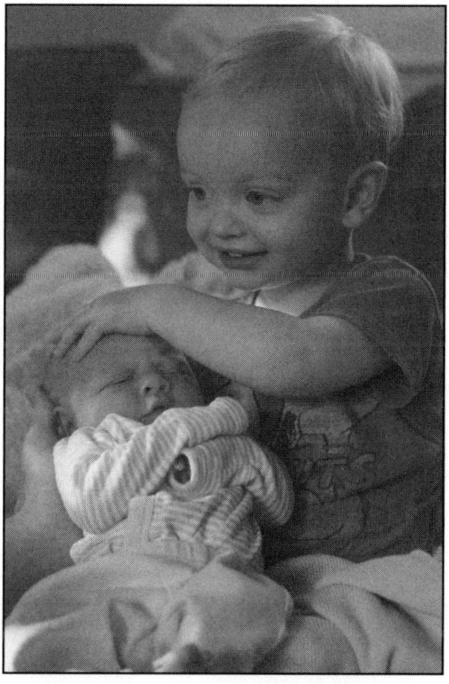

Reagan welcomes his baby sister, Liberty "Libby" Grace.

Owen's Birth Story

When the due date of my son neared, I thought I was completely prepared for his birth. I had read all the books, taken all the classes, and talked to many friends about their birth experiences. I thought the more stories I heard, the better prepared I would be.

My birth plan was to deliver my son as naturally as possible. Ideally, I would spend the early stages of labor at home, drive to the hospital when my contractions were a few minutes apart, and deliver him vaginally with no drugs. Once he was born, I would immediately put him to my breast. However, I am also realistic, and knew there was a possibility that things might not go as planned.

I went into labor four days before my due date. I started having what I thought were Braxton Hicks contractions, but I wasn't certain. About an hour later, there was no doubt that I was having real contractions. I was surprised at how painful they were—and they had only just begun!

Within a few hours I was doubled over in pain, with my contractions coming one right after the other. At that point I knew I needed to get to the hospital. Something wasn't right. I knew I shouldn't be in that much pain that soon.

When we arrived at the hospital, we quickly realized that something was indeed wrong. My son's heart rate was extremely elevated. After unsuccessful attempts to bring it down, I was told that I needed to have a C-section. I honestly have to say that most of that time was (and still is) a complete blur. I remember being scared and in a lot of pain, but mainly focused on getting through each contraction. Once I received the epidural, the pain subsided, and my focus quickly turned to my son and the one thing I thought I wouldn't have to face—a C-section!

Due to the nature of the delivery, it was hours later before I could hold my son in my arms. When I was finally able to hold him, he was very sick so that made breastfeeding a challenge. I knew I should be focusing on the positive, my beautiful baby boy, but I was too sad. I kept replaying everything in my mind, trying to figure out what went wrong. I also think I was in shock that absolutely nothing went as planned—shocked that I could be so healthy, did everything by the book, yet the birth still turned out this way. And I was mostly shocked that the emotional recovery of such an experience could be far more difficult than the physical recovery.

It seems silly that veering from one little plan could cause so much pain. Yet, when you envision something one way and it turns out nothing like that, it takes you by surprise. Although my birth plan did not go as I had "planned," I remind myself that the end result is the same. I have a beautiful, healthy little boy and all that matters is that he is here! The best advice I can offer anyone is to trust ***your*** instincts, be flexible with your birth plan, and be patient with your recovery. One thing is for certain: no one can ever prepare you for how much you will love your child.

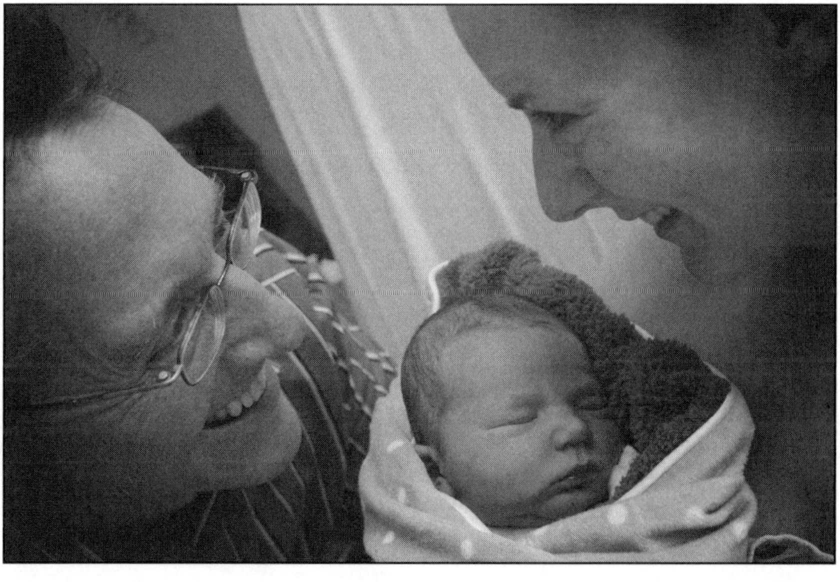

Falling in love with their first son, Owen, Cynthia and Brian treasure these quiet moments following an unexpected emergency C-Birth.

Jasper's Birth Story

My membranes ruptured around 6:00 p.m. on a Friday night. I went to the bathroom and as I was ready to pull up my panties, I began to drip. I assumed that it was extra discharge because I would frequently have extra discharge minutes after going to the bathroom. But I noticed that I kept on leaking so I put on a pad and we went out to eat at Red Robin that night.

After dinner, around 8:15 p.m., as I sat down in the car, a big gush came out between my legs. Instead of going to see a co-worker's band perform, we stayed home. Two of my girlfriends came by to see me as my birthday was that weekend. We watched TV and chatted while I waited for my contractions to progress. Throughout the day I had been very busy at work, and had felt some contractions but thought that I was just a bit overworked. I knew I had to chill out as soon as the day was over. Contractions had been very irregular throughout that day, and continued to be that way Friday night even after my membranes ruptured. I continued to leak throughout the evening. Keith went to bed since we weren't sure how long it would take for my contractions to progress. I stayed up until 1:00 a.m., but the contractions were not progressing or occurring at regular intervals.

I paged my OB and did not hear anything back after an hour. I called the doctor's exchange and at 2:30 a.m., I got a call from the hospitalist OB. She suggested I come in to make sure my membranes had ruptured.

We arrived at the hospital at 3:00 a.m. Five other admissions to L&D had come in that night prior to our arrival. The Ph test strip confirmed that my membranes had ruptured. I was monitored for an hour and a half during my intake and contractions were running about every 5–6 minutes, 1.5 minutes in duration. I was dilated at 1.5 cm. Pitocin was hung at about 6:00 a.m. to advance my contractions.

For the next 3 hours my contractions slowly progressed, from happy face to more grimacing face (based on the pain of contractions chart). The Pitocin dosage was slowly increased. I used the birth ball, and stood at the side of the bed and tried to relax. I brought CDs, but the hospital didn't supply a CD player, so we didn't have music.

At about 9:00 a.m., I was dilated only to 3 cm. More contractions came about every 3–4 minutes and at 11:00 a.m., I was dilated 6 cm and completely thinned out. Thankfully, they lowered the rate of Pitocin as I was not getting much rest in between contractions. I dilated to 8 cm about 45 minutes later, and contractions were coming really heavy. It was harder and harder to relax. Keith said I began to talk in ways I would never talk, that I was making no sense. The last 2 cm were killers. So painful!! I found it hard to move and adjust my position, but I preferred lying on my side at this point. I was difficult to both the nurse and Keith. During the last 2 centimeters of dilation, I felt much more butt pain. I had felt some earlier, when I was at 4–5 cm, but it went away; during this time it was much more intense.

The nurse checked me just after 12:00 noon; she said I had a "lip" she needed to push away, then I'd be ready to push. This "lip-pushing" was not fun. This had to happen during a contraction. I felt like a ketchup bottle that someone slid a knife into to help the ketchup come out easier. Imagine me as the ketchup bottle and the nurse's finger as the knife. As she did that, I felt that Jasper was going to come out right then! With what little might I had left, I prevented myself from pushing. After that I was finally at 10 cm! It took me about 4 or 5 rounds of pushing. I was exhausted. I tried to hold my breath for only a 6-second count like we learned in class, but the team was saying I was not pushing long enough to move the baby. Also, they wanted me to catch my breath so fast between pushes that I felt like I wasn't getting any air in between pushes. I began to cough and gag a little because I wasn't getting my air, but they insisted I needed to go as fast as possible.

It was very difficult, but I finally pushed him out at 12:55 p.m. He was 5 lb, 6 oz and 19 inches long.

Thank you for all your helpful information to make this event successful. I have learned so much more information with you than with my first pregnancy.

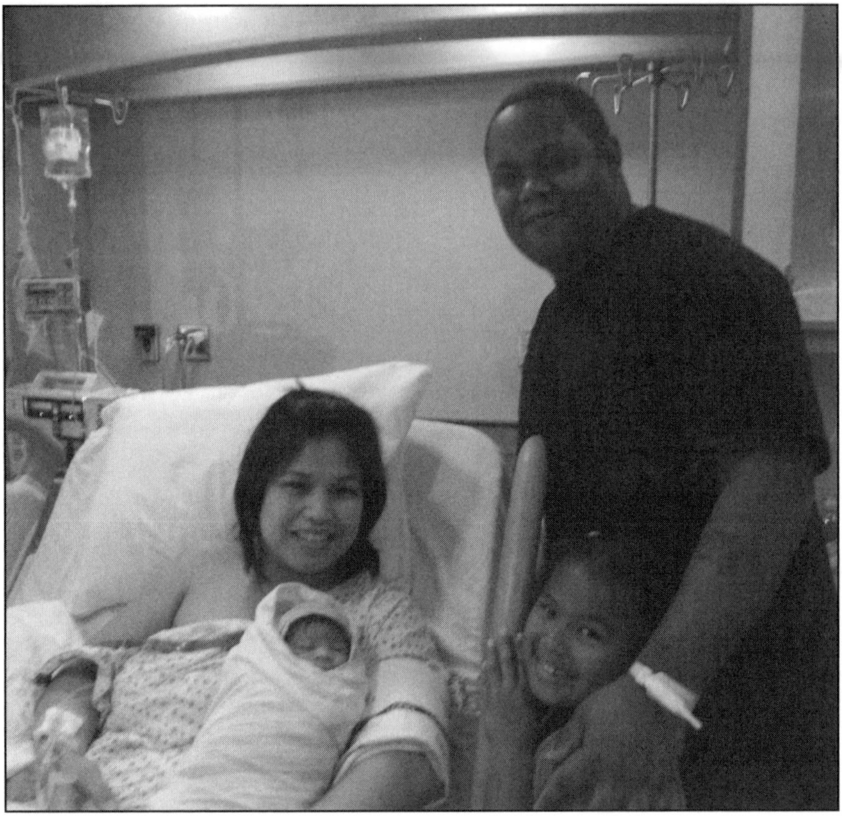

Carrie, Keith and big sister welcome new baby, Jasper.

Sabine and Simone's Birth Stories

Having a C-section with my first pregnancy was not what I planned. But when we found out at 37 weeks that our baby was in a frank breech position and the attempt to change the baby's position using external cephalic version (ECV) was unsuccessful, we shifted gears and began planning for one. Fortunately, our doula was still going to attend our delivery despite the change in delivery route. We modified our birth plan and ended up having the most wonderful birth experience we could have asked for.

Not knowing what sex our baby was, and not announcing our name choices, made us so excited for the birth day. Almost every other detail but those were known ahead of time. The moment the OB held the baby up for my husband to announce her sex, joyfully and with tears in his eyes, was the happiest moment of my life to that point. We filmed the birth and my husband and doula both took photos. I was able to watch in the mirror as Sabine was delivered. With my free hand, I was able to touch her when my husband brought her to me very soon after her birth. Instead of being sent to recovery and my baby sent to the nursery,

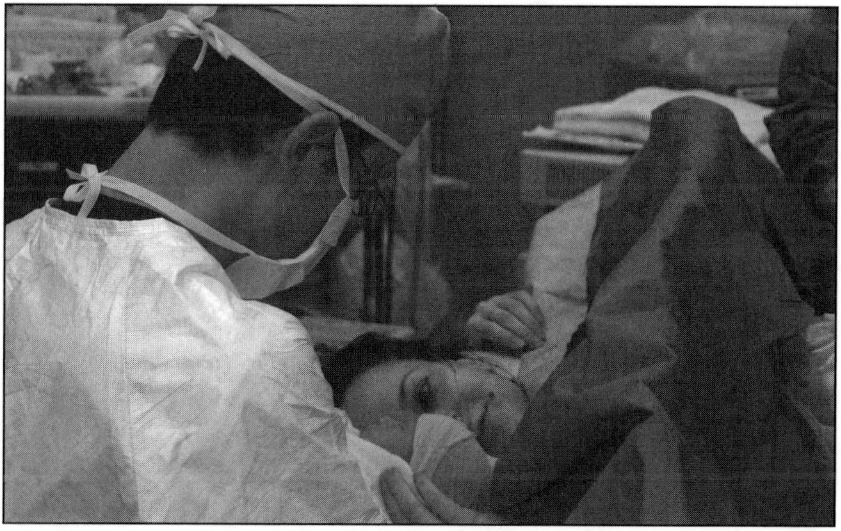

Brian holds Sabine for Dee to see, touch and bond while her surgery is being completed.

our request for the baby to remain with us was granted. After spending some time in the warmer and after only a few essential procedures were done, I breast fed her while in recovery. Soon thereafter, my husband and I gave Sabine her first bath.

After our time in recovery, our baby came with us to our room in the Maternal Infant Unit and she roomed in during our stay. The only time she went to the nursery was for the pediatrician visits, and my husband went along with her. All this time in our room was spent bonding, nursing and sleeping. My husband changed almost every single diaper. By the time we left, we felt in tune with our baby and capable of caring for her on our own. Even as first-time, sleep-deprived parents, we never felt panicky about having her at home with us in those early days.

When I found out I was pregnant with my second child, I was sure I was going to attempt to have a vaginal birth after cesarean. I had already discussed my option for VBAC with my OB before I had my first baby by C-section. She told me that I would be a good candidate for a VBAC given that the reason for cesarean was a breech presentation. I did my research about risks of repeat C-section birth versus VBAC. I decided that if I was really going for it, we would need the support of our doula. I wrote a new birth plan for VBAC. I was hoping to have an unmedicated birth and I requested the use of birthing equipment and alternative pain management techniques such as breathing, distraction, visual imagery and massage. I did not want to be offered pain medication unless I initiated it, and I wanted time to discuss options with my husband and doula in private. I requested that I be able to wear my own clothes and that the room be dimly lit and quiet. We played music that we brought with us. I asked that my IV for antibiotics be heplocked between doses and that I be allowed to consume clear liquids in early labor. I requested that I be able to walk around as much as possible and that continuous fetal monitoring be limited. I wanted to be encouraged to try various labor positions. I requested that I'd like to avoid episiotomy if possible and that methods to reduce the risk of tearing be implemented, including perineal massage, oil, and coaching to slow crowning.

I used the birth mirror and touched her head as it was crowning. My husband once again announced the sex of our baby. Simone was put directly on my bare belly after birth and she was examined by the nursery nurse while lying on my chest. I was able to nurse her before she was taken to the warmer to have essential procedures done. We were able to give our baby her first bath once we were moved to our room in the Maternal Infant Unit. Again, we chose to have our baby room in with us. She was in the nursery only for essential procedures and daily pediatrician exams.

I was very pleased with my birth experience. I found it very comforting to have the relaxed company and support of my doula and husband. My labor and delivery nurse was very respectful of my birth plan requests. When asked about my pain level on the 1 to 10 scale, I found it helpful to give a number lower than it may have been, just so I knew I was not nearing the upper limits. Walking laps around the unit while in early labor helped make the time pass. Humor was another helpful tool we used for pain distraction. I had to tell my husband to stop making me laugh during contractions! I used multiple positions as the contractions grew stronger, from the birthing ball, to sitting on the bed, to standing with my husband's support, to leaning over the bed. My husband massaged my back between contractions. As I entered active labor, I went into "the zone," as my doula called it. Between contractions, I closed my eyes. During contractions, I reached out for my doula and Brian's hands and listened to them talk me through them.

The most difficult part of the delivery was being fully dilated and ready to push, but having to wait for my OB to arrive. Luckily, I made it through that 45 minutes with my doula and husband coaching shallow breaths. They remained very calm and kept telling me I could do it. At one point, I remember looking at my husband and wondering if I could continue on another minute without pushing. He gave me a reassuring look that kept me going until the OB arrived. I was able to hold my own legs with help from my husband and doula. We pulled them way back with each push. I had a wonderful team of cheerleaders including my doula, my husband, the nurse and my OB. Simone's birth was the most rewarding experience of my life.

My husband and I feel very fortunate to have had two special childbirth experiences. I wouldn't change a thing about either birth. Having a birth plan and a team that both advocated for and supported us were the reasons we had such positive experiences despite two very different births.

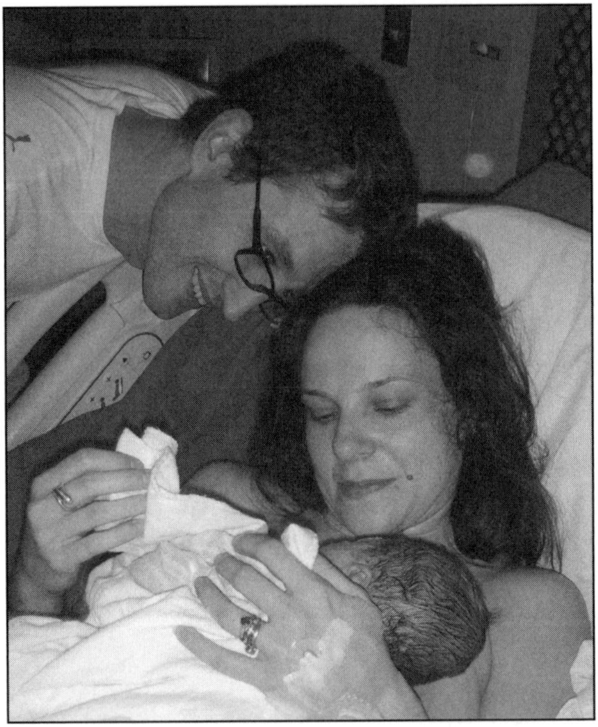

Following a successful VBAC, Brian and Dee welcome another daughter, Simone.

Elena Ivy's Birth Story

I woke with light, crampy contractions around 1:00 a.m. Friday morning. I was able to get some sleep through the cramping from about 4:00 a.m. to noon Friday. I got up and ate lunch. My water must have begun to break around 1:00 p.m. It wasn't the gush I had heard about, but a slow trickle that went on until around 7:00 p.m. Friday. When the leaking continued, I thought I should call the doctor, so I checked in with the nurse around 3:00 p.m. She said if it continued, to call back.

By 4:00 p.m. Dave was home because we knew this would be the night, but wanted to really think about our options and take our time. Our doula Kathy said to call her during her Lamaze class if the water continued to leak but it was such a small amount, it was difficult to tell what was happening. I caught up on my work emails, made some phone calls and took my time deciding to call the doctor back as the leaking continued. I was in a bit of denial, as this was not how I envisioned my labor would begin.

By 6:30 p.m., I had spoken with the doctor on call. She didn't really listen to me. I asked what my options were if my water had broken and she said I had none and would have to be admitted and start on the Pitocin right away. Lovely! I wanted no drugs and to go natural, but she said unless my labor started on its own, without Pitocin, I'd need a C-section within 18 to 24 hours due to "risk of infection" for the baby and me.

I got off the phone and woke Dave up from his nap and told him it was time to head to the hospital. We took our time and did not get there until 8:30 p.m. I took a long shower, put on some light makeup, brushed my hair and even put on some shimmery body lotion. I wanted to feel a bit normal before the patient experience at the hospital. I knew it would be awhile before I would be back at home. I ate a big meal of eggplant Parmesan, some Lucky Charms and a Slim Fast shake. I was carbing up for the big event! I did everything natural I could think of to get contractions going. Dave and I were timing them Friday afternoon but they were so light and sporadic, there was no real pattern.

We got to the hospital and checked in. It was a surreal moment when the doctor (the same one that was on the phone) checked me and confirmed there was no bag anymore, only baby's hair when she checked me. I could not believe all my water was gone. She gave me a semi-concerned smile saying, "Yeah, yeah, we'll need to start the drugs ASAP and admit you so we can get labor going. It's possible to still deliver vaginally, but we are on a time crunch since your water broke at 2:00 p.m."

It was so strange having no options. I understood my birth plan would not be realized. Now the clock was ticking against the 24-hour C-section "deadline" they give you. Mine was for 2:00 p.m. the next day. I had assumed that my minor contractions had dilated me to at least 2 or 2 ½ cm, but I was still only at 1+ cm dilated, and the baby was still high up. The nurses were amazing and knew I wanted natural birth. They encouraged me to wait for our doula Kathy who was getting there at 10:30 p.m. to see if I could go into labor on my own. Nothing happened and when Kathy arrived, we relaxed and hung out and decided to begin the Pitocin around midnight.

By 1:00 a.m. I was having light contractions, no big deal. I brought some fun movies for labor and we put in *Dirty Dancing* first. By the end of *Dirty Dancing*, around 2:30 a.m., I was in active labor. Luckily, I had a nice 3-minute break between contractions during the "I've Had the Time of My Life" finale (I love that movie). I was also able to eat small snacks between contractions up until that point.

The contractions lasted about 1 to 1½ minutes and were 2 to 4 minutes apart. I was able to plow through them with my Lamaze breathing and different focal points. We tried a lot of positions for pain management and comfort. I enjoyed sitting backward on a chair, leaning on some pillows. I also liked resting on the yoga ball, which was on the hospital bed. Lying on my side in the hospital bed was the worst.

From 2:30 a.m. to 6:30 a.m., my contractions got stronger and longer. The night flew by. Elena's heart rate remained steady. Our nurse, Jessica, was amazing and helped a great deal. Kathy helped get me through the toughest ones, and my husband Dave was awesome. Just before 6:00 a.m., our nurse asked if I'd like to be checked for progress. I refused because I did not want to get discouraged. I knew I was making good progress because the contractions were so strong and regular and I could feel the pressure of the baby dropping in my pelvis. The worst part of the labor was from 6:00 a.m. to 7:00 a.m. They turned the Pitocin up and the contractions started rolling one on top of the other. I panicked because it was so excruciating and I could not get a break between them to mentally prepare or physically relax at the beginning of each contraction in order to manage the pain. This was when I asked for the epidural.

I cried and squirmed in pain through a series of 10 to15 contractions that were indescribable. I just could not get control over them. During this time I was checked and was 6 or 7 cm dilated and 90 percent effaced. Yeah! I changed positions to standing and just leaned on Kathy and Dave during the hour waiting for the epidural. I started to gain a little control over the pain with the standing position. Dave kept helping me use the restroom throughout the labor and around 7:30 a.m., I had three of the most powerful contractions ever in the bathroom.

When we left the bathroom I saw that Martha, our anesthesiologist, was there! Wow. What a cool moment. I knew the end of the pain was near. My new nurse, Tricia, helped me through the contractions while I got the epidural and immediately I felt relief from the spinal in the middle of a contraction. Dave and Kathy came back in the room and when I was checked at 8:00 a.m., I was 9½ cm dilated, almost ready to push! I saw my family at 8:30 a.m. and had some time to relax before pushing.

At 9:30 a.m., I was a full 10 and the baby had dropped fully. They called the doctor. The new doctor on call showed up, barely saying a word to me, and we got started.

I started pushing at 10:00 a.m., and Elena was born at 10:40 a.m. The pushing was great. It was amazing to look in the mirror and see her being born. They put her on my chest right away and we had a full 30 or so minutes to bond and feed her before they weighed her and gave her the eye drops. This time with her was so cool. I could not believe it! Except for those 15 or so crazy contractions, it was an amazing labor experience. I was so excited how strong she was through labor and how I was able to handle the whole experience. Wow! 8 pounds 2 ounces, 19 3/4 inches.

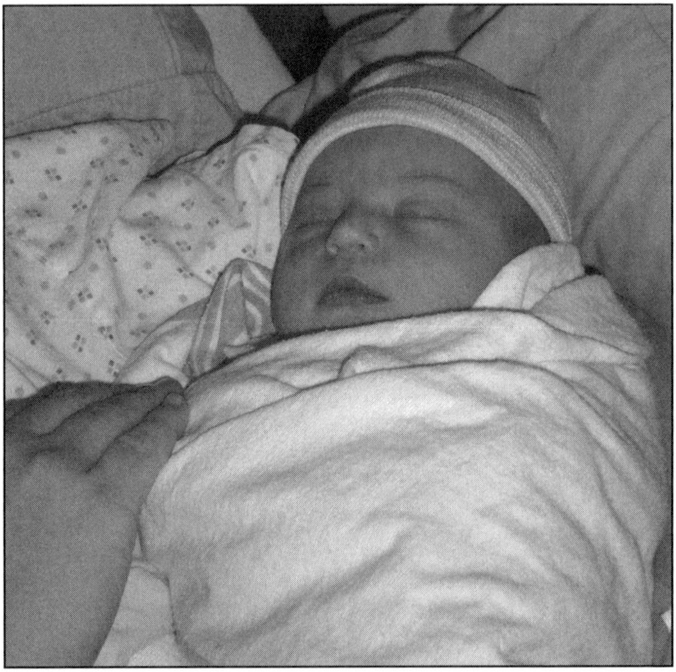

Elena Ivy snuggles in mother Jennifer's arms as her dad, Dave, is close by.

Lucian's Birth Story

During the first six months of our pregnancy, we were under the care of my OB/GYN, a doctor that I had been a patient of for many years and really liked. She is very supportive of natural birthing, and since we had told her we wanted to Lamaze and wanted minimal interventions, we felt very comfortable with her care. However, when we went on the hospital tour, there were so many rules and restrictions; no eating or drinking during labor, the tub was in a completely separate room, and worst of all, they would let the baby stay with us for only an hour after birth before he was whisked away to the nursery. The very idea of being separated from my baby was the deal breaker for me. I knew I wanted to have this baby at home.

At my next OB appointment, I discussed my concerns about the hospital with my doctor. I told her that I wanted to have a home birth and needed to find a qualified midwife. She gave me the name and number of a very highly respected and experienced midwife, and I got in touch with her. I had a lot of confidence in her to begin with, because I had asked around and talked to as many people as possible, and they all said wonderful things about her and that she had been delivering babies "forever." We switched over our care at 30 weeks, with the full support of our OB.

I went into labor at 41 weeks. I labored for about 12 hours before our midwife came to our house; I had been in constant phone contact with her throughout the early stages as she talked to me about what to expect next, what it would feel like and she reassured me that all was proceeding normally. Early on a Saturday morning, she arrived and did an exam, found that I was at three centimeters and that I had some scar tissue on my cervix that was preventing it from dilating further. Our baby was also in an almost posterior position, different from our most recent exam. She broke up the scar tissue on my cervix, and she and my husband helped to turn him. After the scar tissue had been loosened, I dilated almost immediately to four and labor began to pick up. In the early afternoon, after some more intense contractions, I got into the tub when I was at six centimeters. It felt great! It was almost immediate pain relief, and the contractions really went down in intensity. After an hour, I got out of the tub, and labor had slowed significantly, so we did some fast walking up and down, through the living room, kitchen, dining room and bedroom. Later that afternoon, I was getting really tired and ready to have this baby. I had already been in labor for about twenty-four hours at this point, and was ready for it to be over. Our midwife was checking the baby's heart rate frequently to make sure he wasn't getting stressed, and he was fine. She suggested that breaking my water might be the boost we needed to get this show on the road and have a baby before the sun went down. I was apprehensive about how painful it would become, but I was ready to do what I had to do to have this baby. She warned me that if we were to break my water, the contractions were going to get really intense, and that they would come one right after the other, but that it would really get this labor going. I agreed.

She was right! It got intense. I was lying on the living room floor, with my head in my husband's lap. My midwife and husband massaged me during contractions, while I moaned and screamed and shook. My dog and cat came and sat by me as I went through transition. After an hour and a half of really intense contractions, I felt like I had to scramble to my knees, and I did. I had several more contractions on my knees, leaning over our birthing ball, and really, really, really wanted to get back in the tub for the pain relief. Our midwife wanted to see how far along I was before I got back in the tub; we didn't want to slow labor down again now that it was finally happening. She patted me on my back and said, "You're ten" (centimeters dilated). She and my husband sprang into action, topping off the tub with warm water. I was a little stunned that the moment I had been waiting for so long had arrived, and felt a little scared that it was here. She helped me get into the tub, helped me to refocus and calm down. The warm water helped so much! It became almost immediately less painful and the warmth was very soothing and calming. I floated in the tub for a while and let the idea that I had to push this baby out sink in. After awhile my husband got in the tub with me, and being curled up in his arms really helped me to summon the courage to birth our baby.

My midwife had spent so much time talking to me during our prenatal visits about the different stages of labor, and what pushing would be like. She is very proactive about reducing the amount of trauma to the perineum, and she emphasizes that the baby should come out slowly and very controlled to minimize any tearing. I listened to her voice and let her guide me through each contraction. It was the hardest thing in the world not to push when she told me not to, but I'm glad that I didn't push. I delivered him, all 7 lb, 12 oz, without a single tear. I pulled him out of the water myself, and into our arms. Our hands were the first to touch him. It was surreal, watching him come through the blurry water, becoming clearer and clearer as he surfaced. It was beautiful and one of the most powerful experiences of my life.

I am extremely glad that we decided to have our baby at home. We did our research and felt confident that in the hands of an experienced midwife, home birth can be the perfect choice for some families. I wouldn't change a thing about any of our plans or the decisions we made. We are definitely planning a home birth for our next child. And the best part was we got to go to sleep that night in our own bed, both of us snuggled around our new baby.

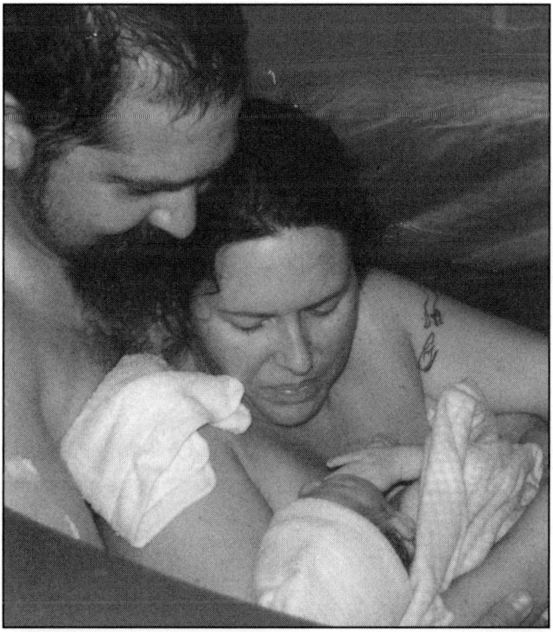

Shannon and Rob welcome their first child, Lucian.

Each of these birth stories is very unique and individual, just like every baby, every mother, every father, every family. All are different and inspiring in their own ways, reflecting many different experiences of birth. I hope that you feel empowered after reading and sharing in these families' stories.

Be sure to write a birth plan that reflects your vision of your baby's birth. Communication is a key. I wish for each of you readers a fulfilling birth experience. At the end of the day, while you hold your precious baby, I want you to reflect on your strengths displayed as you tackled the challenges of labor. Be proud of your accomplishments.

Remember:

When thinking of your life's journey as a person, partner and a parent, there are things that really matter in life. From his book *Life's Greatest Lessons,* Hal Urban writes the following "20 Things That Matter in Life."

Make a copy of these twenty things and place in a location where you can read them daily. I also recommend reading Hal Urban's book. It's very inspirational.

20 Things That Matter in Life

1. Success is more than making money.
2. Life is hard… and not always fair.
3. Life is also fun… and incredibly funny.
4. We live by choice, not by chance.
5. Attitude is a choice—the most important one you'll ever make.
6. Habits are the key to all success.
7. Being thankful is a habit—the best one you'll ever have.
8. Good people build their lives on a foundation of respect.
9. Honesty is still the best policy.
10. Kind words cost little but accomplish much.
11. Real motivation comes from within.
12. Goals are dreams with deadlines.
13. There's no substitute for hard work.
14. You have to give up something to get something.
15. Successful people don't find time—they make time.
16. No one else can raise your self-esteem.
17. The body needs nutrition and exercise—so do the mind and spirit.
18. It's ok to fail—everyone else has.
19. Life is simpler when we know what's essential.
20. Essential # 1 is being a good person.

—Hal Urban
Life's Greatest Lessons

In Summary

I hope you have learned some important lessons in life from reading this book. I especially hope that you will remember the following things:

Trust your body—get in tune with the signals your body is giving you and while sitting still, be amazed at how effortlessly your baby grows in your uterus.

Educate yourself on all your options for pregnancy, birth, and postpartum. Write a birth plan that states your wishes. Share this information with your partner, other support person(s), and your healthcare provider. If your healthcare provider doesn't support your plan, change to one that does. Most midwives are always supportive. Hire a doula so she can support both you and your partner. Remember to ask for what you want… if you don't ask, you will never receive.

Empower yourself… develop the "I can handle it" attitude. Do the positive affirmations. Complete the mindset questions. Getting organized always decreases your stress level.

Compliment yourself. After you give birth, focus on the positive things that occurred during birth and early postpartum period such as the support you received from your partner and/or doula. Make peace with decisions you made during labor that you may have not planned to do. Take time for yourself. Always do the simple things in life for yourself like a manicure, massage, day out with girlfriends or date with your partner. As you hold your beautiful baby close, be amazed by the fact that you had life pass through you and that this little one is growing and thriving on breastmilk, your care and your love. Remember to tell your partner "thank you" for the support you received. Appreciate the loving presence, the tender touch and the many hours of providing comfort measures that your partner brought to the birth experience. This may have been your partner's first time experiencing pregnancy, witnessing birth, and coping with sleep exhaustion. You are both learning together.

Enjoy the little things in life like your baby's first smile, belly laughter, hearing the words "I love you," rocking your precious child to sleep and breathing in your baby's sweet smell. Teach your children your values. Read daily. Pray for wisdom to nurture your beautiful child.

I wish for you a fulfilling pregnancy, birth and postpartum journey. Happy Birthing!

References

Chapter 1

M. Diego, "Maternal Psychological Distress, Prenatal Cortisol and Fetal Weight," *Psychosomatic Medicine* 68:747-753 (2006).

Marshall Sylver, *Passion, Power, and Profit*, Simon, Schuster 1995.

John Gray, *Men Are From Mars, Women Are From Venus*, Harper Collins, 1992.

Chapter 2

Mike Dooley, *Infinite Possibilities*, Atria Books, 2009

Marshall Klaus, *Mothering the Mother-How a Doula Can Help You Have a Shorter, Easier, and Healthier Birth*, Perseus Publisher, 1993.

Chapter 3

G. Carroli and J. Belizan, "Episiotomy for Vaginal Birth" (Cochrane Review) in the *Cochrane Library Issue* 1, Update Software (2001).

W. Sears and M. Sears, *The Birth Book*, Little, Brown and Company, 1994.

Penny Simkin, Janet Whalley, Ann Keppler, *Pregnancy, Childbirth and the Newborn-The Complete Guide*, Meadowbrook Press, 2001

M. Benson, *Obstetrical Pearls: A Practical Guide for the Efficient Resident*, 2nd edition, E.F. Davis Company, 1994.

Chapter 4

Sheila Kitzinger, *The Year After Childbirth*, Charles Scribner's Sons, 1994.

Barbara Harper, *Gentle Birth Choices*, Healing Art Press, 1994.

Chapter 5

Hal Urban, *Life's Greatest Lessons: 20 Things That Matter.*

Chores

- Laundry
- Litterbox
- feeding / pilling mia
- Dishes
- vacuuming
- grocery shopping
- trash / recycling (take out)
- water plants
- mow lawn

Fave foods

- lasagna (no sausage)
- greek yogurt
- Chicken + brocoli casserole
- salads
- minestrone / veggie soups / soup w/ veggies
- anything w/ Quinoa
- Quiche (no pork)
- egg casserole (no pork)
- mexican food

Your Mindset for Postpartum

Your Mindset on Becoming a Parent

Full Circle Childbirth Consultants, Inc.
Birth Plan

Mother's Name ____________________ **Support Person** ____________________

Doctor ____________________ **Due Date** ____________________

First Stage

Positions

Walking	____
Standing	____
Rocking	____
Lunge	____
Sitting	____
Birth Ball	____
Lying Down	____
Back of Bed	____

Comfort Measures

Showers	____
Massage	____
Hot Packs	____
Cold Packs	____
Music	____

Phone

Incoming calls	____
Only call out	____

Fluids

Ice Chips	____
Ice Pops	____
Juice	____
I.V.	____

Monitor

Continuous	____
Intermittent	____
External	____
Internal	____

Medication

None	____
Narcotics	____
Epidural	____

Second Stage

Positions

Squatting	____
Side Lying	____
Semi Sitting	____
Hands & Knees	____

Perineal Care

Perineal Massage	____
Warm Compresses	____
Episiotomy	____

I (we) feel strongly about the following:

Glossary

Abruptio Placenta: This is when the placenta separates from the wall of the uterus before the baby is born. This puts the mother and baby in danger and requires an emergency C-Birth.

Amniotic Fluid: Fluid found in the amniotic sac that surrounds the baby in utero.

Amniotic Sac: Thin-walled bag that contains amniotic fluid, baby, placenta and umbilical cord. Also known as the bag of water.

Analgesics: Another word for pain relievers. Common analgesics used in labor are narcotics like Stadol or Nubain.

Apgar Score: Test that assesses a newborn's well-being at one and five minutes after birth. It rates the skin color, baby's heart rate, reflexes, muscle tone and breathing rate.

Birthing Center: Home-like setting which gives couples an alternative to a hospital birth. Usually staffed with certified midwifes.

Birth Canal: The passageway for the baby. Another name for the vagina.

Birth Plan: An excellent communication tool that contains a couple's written birth desires and concerns. It should be shared with the healthcare provider, doula and nursing staff.

Bloody Show: Blood-tinged mucous that passes out of the vagina during labor, which indicates the cervix (neck of the uterus) is dilating and/or effacing.

Braxton-Hicks Contractions: Intermittent contracting of the uterus which occurs throughout the pregnancy, most noticed during the last trimester. This contracting doesn't cause any cervical changes.

Breech Presentation: Position of the baby in the uterus when the presenting part is the baby's buttocks or feet instead of the head down position.

Catecholamines: These are sympathomimetic "fight or flight" hormones that are released by the adrenal glands in response to stress. When in labor, if a mother feels stressed, her body will release these hormones causing her labor to slow down or stop.

Cesarean Birth: Surgical delivery of a baby through an abdominal incision.

Cervix: The opening or neck of the uterus. The cervix is approximately 1½ inches long, thick and firm. During the last 4 weeks of pregnancy, the cervix becomes soft (ripen) and begins to thin (effacement). This thinning is measured in percentage with 0 percent long and thick and 100 percent effaced is completely thinned.

Contractions: Rhythmic tightening and shortening of the uterine muscle, working to dilate and efface the cervix and push the baby through the birth canal.

Cord Prolapse: An emergency situation in which the umbilical cord slips out of the uterus in front of the baby, blocking all blood flow to the baby. An emergency C-Birth is required.

Crowning: The appearance of the baby's head on the mother's perineum as it comes through the birth canal.

Dilation: In regards to pregnancy – dilation is the opening of the cervix of the uterus. This is measured in centimeters…completely closed cervix is 0 centimeters - completely opened cervix is 10 centimeters.

Doula: An experienced woman who provides continuous physical and emotional support for the laboring mother.

Effacement: The thinning of its walls and shortening of the cervix as it stretches and widens by the pressure of the baby's head (or presenting part) as the contractions intensify.

Electronic Fetal Monitoring (EFM): An electronic fetal monitoring device that monitors and records the fetal heart tones.

Engaged: This refers to when the baby's head descends into the pelvis and may occur several weeks before the onset of labor.

Epidural: Frequently used form of anesthesia during childbirth to relieve pain. Excellent form of anesthesia used for C-Births, allowing the mother to stay awake during the surgery.

Episiotomy: Incision that is made on the perineum (between the vaginal opening down toward the rectum) to enlarge the birth canal.

False labor: Irregular tightening (contracting) of the pregnant uterus that can increase in frequency, intensity and duration but doesn't cause any cervical changes. Usually these contractions will not have all three (longer, stronger, closer together) characteristics at the same time and may come and go for hours or days without changing the cervix to dilate or efface.

Fetal Distress: Occurs when the fetus isn't receiving enough oxygen from the placenta, causing the fetus's heart rate to drop to a very low rate or rise to a dangerously high rate, putting the baby into distress. Cord compression is one reason. Immediate delivery is sometimes required while at other times, changing the mother's position and giving her oxygen will resolve the distress by relieving the compression on the cord.

Fetal Scalp Electrode: An internal monitoring device that is placed under the skin of the fetus's scalp during labor to obtain a more accurate monitoring of the fetus' heartbeat.

Fontanel: The "soft spots" are areas between the bones of the baby's skull that feel soft when touched. These soft spots allow the baby's head to elongate or mold in order to fit through the birth canal and also allow for the baby's brain to grow throughout the next 2 years of life. Once the baby is approximately 18-24 months of age, the bones in the skull will permanently fuse.

Forceps: These two metal blades are placed on each side of the baby's head in the birth canal and are used to assist in helping a woman give birth. The mother must push as the healthcare provider guides the baby out.

Fundus: Refers to the top of the uterus.

Group B Strep: This group B streptococcus infection is common bacteria found in 10-35 percent of women's lower intestines and/or in the vagina which is usually harmless to healthy adults. If this bacterium is in the vagina at the time of birth, it may be passed to the baby when born vaginally. If the baby contracts this bacterium, he can become very ill. Most pregnant women are tested at 36 weeks and if the culture is positive for the bacteria, treatment with antibiotics will be started in early labor.

Induced labor: Labor that is artificially started with either Pitocin, synthetic oxytocin, or rupturing the amniotic sac is called "to be induced." There are many medical reasons that warrant inductions but should not be done just for convenience of the parents or the healthcare provider.

Labor: Term used in pregnancy that describes the onset of the uterus muscles contracting in a rhythmic pattern that causes dilation and effacement of the cervix.

Lightening: Term used describing when the baby is "dropping" down into the pelvis after 36 weeks, getting ready for labor.

Lochia: Vaginal discharge that occurs after delivery of the placenta, may last up to 40 days postpartum. First few days, lochia is a bright-red, bloody discharge—like a heavy menstrual period flow in amount, following a few days to weeks. This discharge will be lighter in amount and pinker in color, then may continue for 40 days with a whitish discharge. It should never smell foul.

Meconium: First stool passed by the newborn. It is thick, black and very sticky in consistency.

Mindset: Refers to your current state of thinking.

Molding: The natural process by which the baby's bones of the scalp overlap each other to allow the head to "mold" into a better shape to fit through the pelvis during birth.

Mucous Plug: Thick mucous that is in the cervix of the uterus and is often noticed by the mother up to several weeks before onset of labor.

Non-Stress Test: A non-invasive evaluation of the response of the fetus to natural contractions. It is commonly done in the healthcare provider's office, especially if the mother is past her due date.

Oxytocin: A hormone that is produced in the pituitary gland that causes uterine contractions as well as stimulates the flow of breast milk. This hormone is also called the "love hormone" because when a person feels loved, is touched or sexually stimulated, a surge of oxytocin is released, giving the person a sense of excitement, calm, peace and of being loved.

Perineum: Area of the skin located between the vagina to the rectum.

Pitocin: A synthetic oxytocin which is used to stimulate the uterine contractions.

Placenta: Embryonic tissue that forms an organ that is responsible for nutrition and removal of waste for the fetus during pregnancy. The umbilical cord connects the placenta to the fetus.

Placenta Previa: The condition occurs when the placenta grows low in the uterus, covering the cervical opening, making it impossible for the fetus to be born vaginally.

Postpartum: Period of time immediately after birth of the baby up to one year.

Postpartum Depression: Depression that occurs shortly after childbirth up to one year postpartum. A few symptoms are sadness, crying, unable to sleep, decreased appetite, lack of interest in baby or feelings of harming your baby. Treatment needs to be started as soon as possible.

Post Term: When a pregnancy continues longer than 42 weeks gestation.

Preterm Labor: When labor begins before 37 weeks gestation, babies are at higher risk of having health issues, especially respiratory problems.

PROM: Acronym used for premature rupture of membrane.

Prostaglandin gel or cream: Medication commonly used to ripen the cervix before labor needs to be induced.

Ruptured Membranes: Refers to when the fluid-filled amniotic sac that surrounds the fetus breaks.

Shoulder Dystocia: Occurs at the time of delivery when the baby's shoulder gets caught on the mother's pubic bone.

Station: This describes the location of the top of the baby's head in relationship to the mother's pelvis. Measured at the top of mother's pelvis : -4, -3, -2, -1, 0 station, +1, +2, +3, +4 —at which time the baby's head is in the mother's perineum. Also known as crowning.

Term: Refers to a pregnancy that goes to 40 weeks gestation. Preterm is when the pregnancy ends before 37 weeks; post-term is when the pregnancy goes longer than 42 weeks gestation.

Timing Contractions: Timing duration of contractions starts with the beginning of the uterus tightening until the uterus is relaxed…measured in seconds. Timing frequency starts by timing the beginning of one contraction until the beginning of the next contraction.

Transverse: Refers to the position of the fetus in the uterus. The fetus is lying horizontally across the uterus instead of vertical.

Umbilical Cord: Cord that connects the fetus to the placenta in utero. It has two arteries and one vein and is buried in Wharton's jelly and is responsible for providing nutrition to the fetus and removing waste.

Uterus: Female reproductive organ that houses the fetus during pregnancy.

Vacuum Extractor: This medical assisted device is used to help guide the fetus out of the birth canal by attaching a soft suction cup to the top of the fetus's head.

VBAC: This abbreviation means - Vaginal Birth After Cesarean

Vernix : This is the cheesy white substance that covers and protects the fetus's skin in utero from the amniotic fluid.

RECOMMENDED READING

Books on Pregnancy, Childbirth, Breastfeeding and Postpartum

Note: Bold type indicates my favorite books I recommend for parents.

Pregnancy and Childbirth

***Pregnancy, Childbirth and the Newborn* – Janet Whalley, Penny Simkin & Keppler**
***Ina May Gaskin's Guide to Childbirth* – Ina May Gaskin**
Thinking Woman's Guide to a Better Birth – Henci Goer
Active Birth – Janet Balaskas
***The Birth Partner* – Penny Simkin**
***The Birth Book* – Dr. William and Martha Sears, RN, IBCLC**
Trust your Body! Trust your Baby! – Andrea Frank Henkart
Easing Labor Pain – Adrienne Lieberman
Good Birth, Safe Birth – Dianna Korte and Roberta Scaer
A Child is Born – Lennart Nilsson
***The Complete Book of Pregnancy and Childbirth* – Shelia Kitzinger**
Birth Over Thirty-five – Shelia Kitzinger
Having Twins – Elizabeth Noble

Postpartum and Baby Care

***The First Year After Childbirth* – Shelia Kitzinger**
***The Baby Book* – Dr. William and Martha Sears, RN, IBCLC**
The Discipline Book – Martha Sears, William Sears, MD
***Touchpoints* – T. Barry Brazelton, MD**
Keys to Becoming a Father – William Sears, MD
Getting Organized for Your New Baby – Maureen Bard
Mayo Clinic Book of Pregnancy & Baby's First Year – Robert V. Johnson
Welcoming Your Second Baby – Vicki Lansky

The Fussy Baby – Dr. William Sears
***The Happiest Baby on the Block* – Harvey Karp**

Breastfeeding

Nursing Mother's Companion – Kathleen Huggins
The Womanly Art of Breastfeeding – LLLI

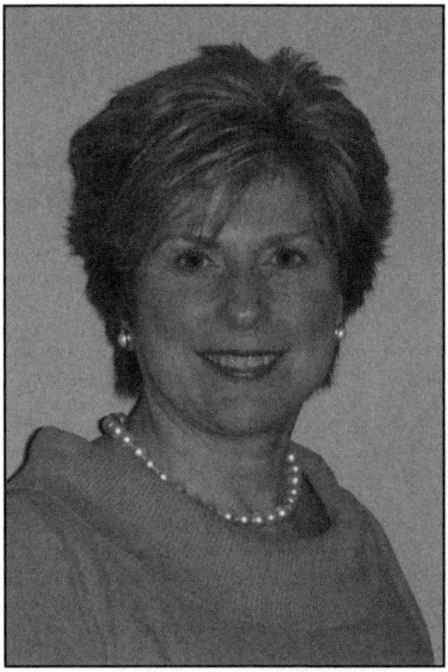

About the Author

Kathy Malone Stewart has worked as a certified pediatric nurse practitioner for over thirty years, graduating from Virginia Commonwealth University/Medical College of Virginia in 1979. She works part-time in a private pediatric office as a CPNP and lactation consultant (IBCLC), giving her time to pursue her other interests, which are teaching Lamaze classes, working with couples as their birth or postpartum doula (DONA certified), training other women to become doulas and lecturing on empowerment issues. Her motivation for writing this book is to help couples create a meaningful birth plan and to empower them to take an active role in their preparation for birth as well as helping them to effectively communicate with their healthcare provider, doula, and nursing staff.

In 1996, Kathy incorporated her company, Full Circle Childbirth Consultants, to expand her mission from offering prenatal education to providing birth and postpartum services as well as coordinating and training women to become DONA (Doulas of North America) approved birth or postpartum doulas. Full Circle also develops educational programs for continuing education credits on a variety of topics including breastfeeding, comfort measures for the laboring patient, doula support and several pediatrics issues like bedwetting and attention deficit disorder (ADHD).

Kathy is active with the Richmond area Virginia chapter of NAPNAP (National Association of Pediatric Nurse Associates/Practitioners) where she has served as program chairperson and served as the 2009-2010 Virginia chapter president. She is the proud mother of two adult sons.